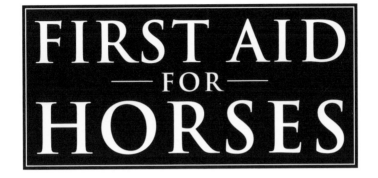

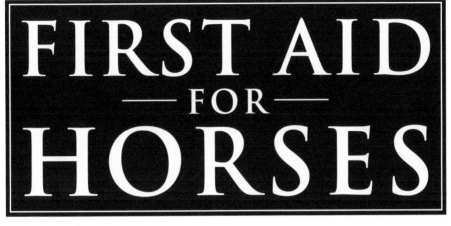

FIRST AID
—FOR—
HORSES

HOW TO COPE WITH INJURY AND ILLNESS

KAREN COUMBE
MA Vet MB CertEP MRCVS

J. A. Allen
LONDON

British Library Cataloguing in Publication Data
A catalogue record for this book is available from the British Library

ISBN-10: 0-85131-780-4
ISBN-13: 978-0-85131-780-9

Published by J. A. Allen & Co. Ltd. 2000
An imprint of Robert Hale Ltd., Clerkenwell House,
45–47 Clerkenwell Green, London ECIR OHT

Reprinted 2001
Reprinted 2003 (twice)
Reprinted 2006

Designed by Judy Linard
Colour separation by tenon & Polert Colour Scanning Ltd.
Printed in China by Midas Printing International Ltd.

CONTENTS

ACKNOWLEDGEMENTS

I would like to thank my family, all my colleagues, clients, students and above all the horses for enabling this book to happen. I am particularly grateful to those who have allowed me to use their pictures, particularly Dr P. D. Clegg, Mr D. C. Knottenbelt, Dr T. S. Mair, Dr A. G. Matthews, Prof. I. G. Mayhew, Dr W. Rosenkrantz, Dr R. K. W. Smith, Dr J. F. Pycock and Dr C. M. Riggs. I also want to thank Louise Harvey for proof-reading and *Horse and Hound* magazine for persuading me that writing is a good idea!

INTRODUCTION

What is first aid?

First aid is the immediate management of any illness or injury and can be crucial in minimising the harm done after an accident. For straightforward injuries, basic first aid may be all that is required. For more major damage, first aid is still important to limit the primary damage, reduce complications and help in producing a full recovery as rapidly as possible.

This guide provides information on this essential first treatment after illness or injury and when it is necessary. It will not replace the need to call your vet, but will help you to recognise problems before they become critical. My aims are to give you an indication of when to seek veterinary advice and also to provide constructive suggestions as to what can be done whilst you are waiting for your vet to arrive. I hope you do not need to use it too often! The idea is to answer the frequently asked questions that a vet has to deal with when on emergency call. Some will be true emergencies and others will not. The purpose of this book is to help you distinguish genuine emergencies and know what to do once you have recognised that a problem exists.

In the event of an accident, everyone in the vicinity is liable to give you advice, much of it conflicting. What appears as a catastrophe when it involves your own horse, will be much more straightforward to a vet who is accustomed to dealing with such injuries. It is best to ask the expert. By discussing the problem with your veterinary surgeon, an apparent crisis may be resolved with some simple first aid advice and reassurance.

The most important item in a first aid kit is your list of essential telephone numbers. At the top of this list should be the contact number for your vet.

Advice regarding genuine emergencies is available on a 24-hour basis from all veterinary practices.

Two very important points are:

- The best person to talk to the vet initially is the person who knows most about the horse's present state. If you have not actually seen the horse yourself, you cannot possibly explain accurately what is wrong! As a vet, there is nothing more frustrating than discussing a potentially serious problem at third hand.

- Try to give the vet as much notice as you can, although this is obviously not possible in a true emergency. If you are worried about a wound or something similar, try to talk to your vet early in the morning, so that a visit can be planned for that day if necessary. Your vet may be somewhat less sympathetic if the injury has been present for several days before you decide to ring, late in the afternoon, after that yard or area has already been visited for the day.

You should aim to develop a good relationship with your veterinary surgeon, so that you can approach him or her easily for help. It is far better to seek professional advice than to take the advice, however well meant, of amateurs.

1. WHAT IS NORMAL FOR YOUR HORSE?

Routine, regular observation of all horses under your care is the best way to prevent problems. It is easy enough to recognise when a horse is really ill, but are you sure you know when he is feeling just less than one hundred per cent? For example, can you (or could anyone) tell if your horse has a headache? It can be very hard to recognise when a horse is a little bit off colour. The more that you know what he is usually like, the easier it is to tell if something is wrong. The simple way of remembering what to look for is to think of ABC, meaning **appearance**, **behaviour** and **condition**. Check each of these in turn and routine observation will become second nature!

A responsible horse owner should be able to measure their horse's temperature, pulse and respiratory rate. It is a good idea to check the normal values for your own horses so that you will be able to tell what is unusual for them.

The normal temperature for an adult horse is 37° to 38°C or 100° to 101° F.

The normal pulse should be between 35 to 42 beats per minute.

The normal respiratory rate at rest is between 8 to 20 breaths per minute.

Taking the temperature

Special veterinary thermometers can be purchased, although a human thermometer will work. The ideal is an easy-to-read digital thermometer. If you use a glass thermometer make sure the mercury is shaken down to the end of the thermometer before you start, as it will not record a lower reading accurately if the mercury is at the top of the scale.

When taking a horse's temperature it is important to stand to the side to avoid being kicked, and to lift up the tail carefully

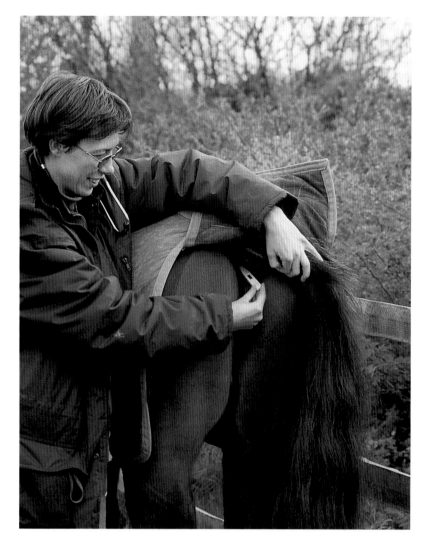

- A horse's temperature is measured in the rectum. Grease the measuring end with some lubrication, such as petroleum jelly (e.g. Vaseline®) or saliva. It is safest to have someone steadying the horse's head and reassuring him. Stand to one side of the rear of the horse, run your hand over the quarters and then grasp the base of the tail firmly. Gently lift it and then carefully insert the thermometer into the anus. Keep hold of the tail so the horse does not clamp it down, but also hang on to the thermometer so that you do not lose it. Stay to the side and be careful to avoid being kicked. Leave the thermometer inserted for about a minute, making sure you tilt it against the wall of the rectum, rather than in the centre of a ball of faeces. Then gently remove it, wipe it clean with a tissue or cotton wool and read it. Afterwards clean it with cold water and disinfectant.

- A slightly increased temperature is not usually serious and is normal after exercise.
- A high temperature (much more than 40°C or 102.5°F) is potentially serious. It suggests that the horse has some form of illness, most likely a viral or bacterial infection. You should contact your vet for advice.
- A very low temperature suggests the horse is not well and may even be going into a state of shock.

Measuring the pulse

The best place to feel a horse's pulse is where the facial artery passes under the jaw. Make sure the head is still and the horse is not eating when you do this. The horse's resting pulse is slow, so it can be difficult to detect on a moving target. Practise finding your horse's pulse after he has been working, when it will be stronger and therefore more obvious.

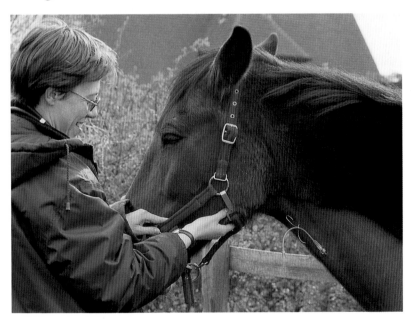

A good place to measure a horse's pulse is by feeling the artery as it runs over the angle of the jaw, as shown

- To find the pulse, run your fingers along the bony lower edge of the jaw. The pulsing artery will be felt as a tubular structure. If you press this lightly against the jaw with the flat of your first three fingers, you will feel the pulse. Count the number of beats in fifteen seconds and multiply by four to get the pulse rate per minute.
- A horse's pulse will increase with exercise, excitement, a high temperature or pain.
- If you cannot feel the pulse, feel for the heart beat on the left side of the lower chest, where the girth would go, just behind the elbow.

Measuring the respiratory rate

To check this, either hold a hand close to the horse's nostrils to feel each breath, or count flank movements. On a cold day you will be able to see each time he exhales.

- The respiratory rate increases with exercise, pain and high temperature, as well as with respiratory disease itself. It is worth noting that a horse usually has around three heart beats to every one breath. This ratio stays about the same with exercise, but not with disease. Any significant change should be taken seriously. A horse with a severe breathing problem will have only one heart beat for three breaths or even worse. When horses have difficulty in breathing they flare their nostrils and the whole of their flanks will lift up and down with the extra respiratory effort.

Other signs to look for

- **The skin** should be supple and loose. It should spring back into shape immediately after pinching. If it remains 'tented', this suggests dehydration. A horse has to be very dehydrated for obvious skin tenting to be noticeable. The best place to look for skin tenting is just above the eyes.
- **The mucous membranes** around the eye and on the gums should be a healthy salmon pink colour apart from the occa-

sional horse that has pigmented gums. With serious illness, such as jaundice, the membranes change colour. It is possible to check the circulation by measuring the 'capillary refill time'. This can be done by pressing a pink area of the gums. This should blanche with pressure and then return to normal within three seconds. A delay suggests a circulatory problem such as shock.

- **Sweating** for no obvious reason implies something is wrong, e.g. the horse may be in pain.

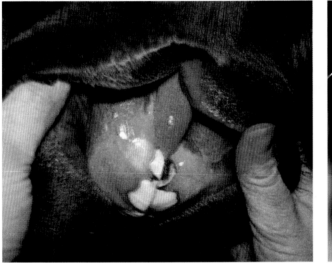

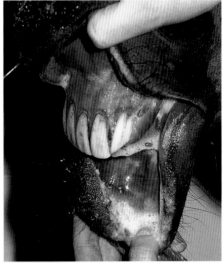

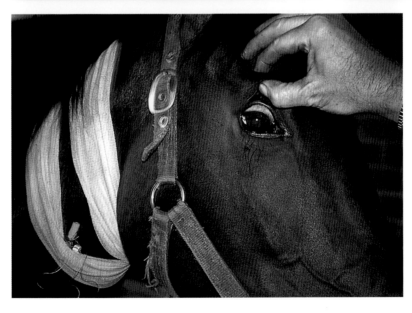

Top left: Checking the membrane colour of the gums; the black pigmentation is normal and *not* a sign of disease

Left: Checking the mucous membranes around the eye. In this case they are very yellow and the horse is jaundiced

Above: Here the horse's gums are a dark purple-blue colour as a result of shock

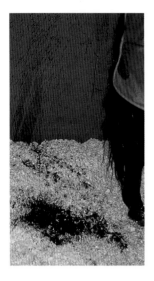

Always look in the stable for normal droppings. Watch out for staining of the walls and bedding, as here with diarrhoea

- **The droppings** should be monitored. Loose droppings or diarrhoea are a cause for concern. Equally, you should be worried if a horse has passed fewer droppings than normal as this may be an indication of constipation or colic.
- **Urine** should also be checked. It is normal for a horse's urine to be a very cloudy yellow colour, but this can range from a pale yellow to a more brownish colour. If there is a change in colour, and particularly if the urine appears red, you should be concerned. Similarly, if a horse is repeatedly straining to pass urine, this suggests there is some pain somewhere. Passing urine more frequently is less likely to be serious but still suggests something may be wrong.
- **Appetite:** Ponies are almost always hungry, so if they stop eating it usually means they are ill. Horses are fussier and will stop eating if they are excited or otherwise disturbed. In particular, very fit animals can be surprisingly picky eaters. You should know what your individual horse's appetite is like. For many horses being off their food is the *biggest* clue that they are unwell, while others are fussy feeders and will go off their feed for no real reason.
- **Thirst:** Horses normally drink 5 to 10 gallons (approximately 20 to 45 litres) of water a day, but this varies with the individual horse, the weather, the work they are doing and the moisture content of the rest of their diet.

If a horse appears dull and does not want to eat, there is likely to be something wrong

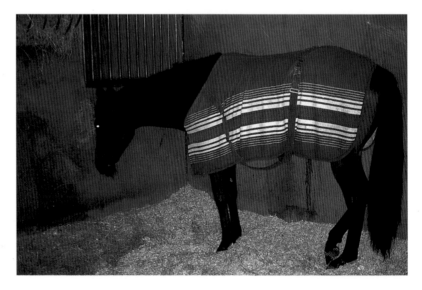

16

- **Mental state:** If a horse appears unusually dull or excited something is wrong.
- **Lameness:** It will be obvious to anybody when a horse is very lame, i.e. it cannot stand on one leg. However, subtle lameness is much harder to appreciate. If you are unsure if your horse is lame, it is best to ask someone to trot the horse away from you and then back towards you on the end of a lead rope with his head held loosely so you can watch it move. A horse that is lame in front will lift his head up as the lame leg hits the ground. The head then nods down as the sound leg hits the ground. Hindlimb lameness can be

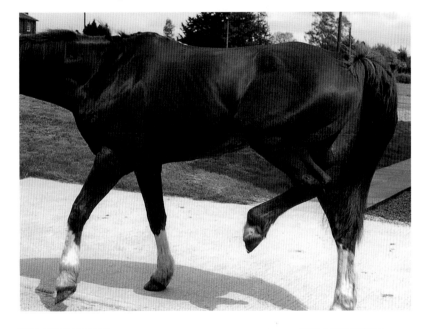

Left: This horse has an obviously abnormal gait, which looks like an odd lameness. This is a result of stringhalt, a nervous condition that is affecting the left hind here

Below: How to tell when a horse is lame on a front leg

THE SOUND HORSE

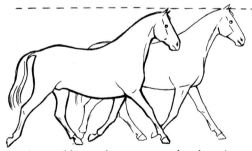

A sound horse shows an even head carriage

THE LAME HORSE

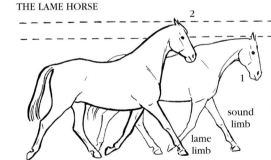

sound limb

lame limb

The lame horse nods as the sound front leg falls (1) and raises its head as the lame limb meets the ground (2).

17

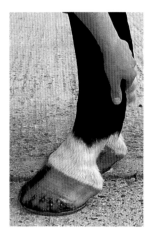

Above: Feeling for digital pulses

Right: A horse or pony that does not try to stand up when a stranger approaches is usually unwell. This pony had such severe laminitis that it found it too painful to stand

harder to spot, but it is easier to see as a horse trots away from you. The hip on the painful lame side appears to rise and fall more obviously as the horse tries to avoid taking weight on that leg.

- **Digital pulses:** If a foot problem is present, a stronger than normal digital pulse may be felt where the artery runs over the fetlock. This happens because of the change in blood flow to the foot and will be more obvious on the affected foot. Compare the different feet. If an abscess or some other foot problem is developing, it may cause a more pronounced pulse to be present. If you find a pounding digital pulse in more than one foot, the most likely cause is laminitis.

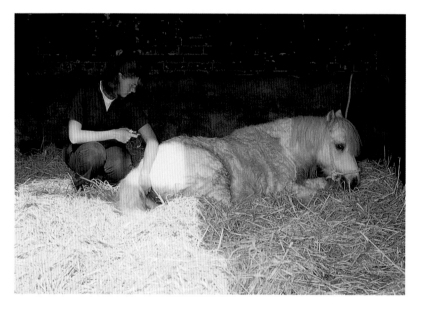

Once you know your own horse, you can usually tell if he is unwell.

2. WHAT SHOULD A FIRST AID KIT INCLUDE?

Anyone who looks after a horse should have some kind of first aid kit available in case of emergencies. With luck, you may never need it, but having it to hand is reassuring. It is important to replace anything you use straightaway because it may be required again in the future. Always have a travelling first aid kit with you when you and your horse are away from home. It is pointless having a comprehensive kit back at the stable yard and nothing with you during a competition. The best option is to have a proper first aid kit back at base and a small travelling first aid box. What you put in each kit rather depends on your own requirements and how accident-prone you and your horse are!

You will need a good **antiseptic**, since the sooner an injury can be cleaned the better. A suitable non-irritant solution can be obtained from your vet. Some commercial antiseptics may be an irritant, as will any antiseptic used at the wrong concentration. In an emergency, use warm salt water (a teaspoon of salt to 1 pint or 0.5 litre of clean water works well). If there is no water available, moist **baby wipes** can be useful for cleaning off superficial dirt especially in a travelling first aid box. However, a wipe is no substitute for thoroughly flushing the dirt out of a wound by hosing it or using a large bag of saline to flush it out.

Everyone includes **wound ointment** and **powder** in a first aid kit but it is questionable whether they are worth having as they are not very effective at controlling infection. They may even seal dirt in, so when they are used it is important to clean any wound thoroughly first otherwise problems may arise.

One special plea from a vet: only use water, antiseptic, wound gel and bandages prior to a vet's examination. It is impossible to check any wound covered with coloured spray or similar! Wound gels (such as Intrasite gel® produced by Smith & Nephew, Nu-gel® from Johnson & Johnson and Derma Gel® from Maximilian Zenho/Equine America) are ideal for first aid. Such soluble gels work very well to keep a wound clean and moist. They are thought to help reduce the bacteria present and may speed healing.

Wound ointments, powders and aerosols are useful as a temporary measure for small cuts. It is justifiable to have wound powder with fly repellent in it to apply to wounds in summer to keep the flies away.

Cotton wool is vital for all first aid kits. A thick roll can also act as bandage padding. When moistened with water, cotton wool is useful for cleaning up everything.

Every first aid kit should include plenty of dressings. You should always have in stock the following:

- **Gamgee** is basically cotton wool sandwiched between gauze. It is worth having plenty of this as it may be essential in an emergency to provide support for an injured leg. It may also be used as a pad to put pressure on a wound, ideally over a non-adhesive dressing. You will need strong **scissors** to cut gamgee.
- **Cotton stretch bandage**, e.g. K band® or a **crepe bandage**, is necessary to hold gamgee in place. I find the 7.5 cm width is best for horses. Many other useful **elastic conforming bandages** are available. Ask your vet which they recommend as there is a great variation in quality and price. Avoid old-fashioned, white, open-weave bandage because it has no stretch. Never stretch a bandage too tightly. Remember, if a leg swells, any dressing will become uncomfortable and start to pinch. If in any doubt, take the dressing off and get expert help. Do not just leave the problem to settle down as a bad bandage can do more harm than the wound it covers.
- **Adhesive bandages** are used to hold other dressings together. You can buy them in both wide and narrow sizes, and a good first aid kit will have both. They help to waterproof a dressing

as well as holding it in position. Such bandages may be expensive. A cheaper alternative is **sticky tape**, such as PVC electrical insulating tape. This will not look as smart but it will hold a temporary dressing in place, which is what first aid is all about. I would suggest a wide (10 cm) and a narrow (2 cm) roll of tape as they are useful for taping all sorts of things together in an emergency.

• **Non-stick dressing pads** are essential to put directly over a wound. When removed, they do not disturb the blood clot over a wound. There are many wound dressings on the market, all designed specifically to help a wound to heal. Again, ask your vet which they recommend.

• **A poultice** is a special dressing which is applied (usually warmed) to increase the local blood supply. The traditional idea is that this 'draws out' infection, and although scientific evidence to prove this may be limited, it can be helpful. 'Animalintex®' is chemical impregnated gauze which can be used to great effect. Kaolin poultices are also useful, and can be applied cold to reduce inflammation. When applying hot poultices, be careful not to scald the skin. Skin wounds do not respond well to repeated poulticing, as, with time, the edges of the wound become soft and will die back. A poultice is good for first aid, but if the problem is not better in 48 hours, consult your veterinary surgeon. Poultices are perfect first aid for foot injuries, such as hoof abscesses, but they are never a substitute for proper cleaning, particularly with skin wounds.

• **Cold bandages** are useful in a travelling first aid kit to treat injuries such as sprained tendons. Research has shown that immediately cooling the leg and providing a support dressing can reduce damage and help healing. Cold bandages are therefore worth having, especially for point-to-pointers and eventers. It will save that panic raid on the beer tent for ice or the rush around to find a bag of frozen peas, both of which are traditional first aid for such injuries. Some of these cold bandages need to be kept in the freezer before use, e.g. the Bonner bandage®. The most modern types release chemical cooling agents when they are taken out of their packet and are very convenient.

Please note that the bandage materials mentioned throughout are given purely as examples and relate to those routinely used in my veterinary practice.

A first aid kit should always include a clean **bucket** and ideally a **bowl** as well. If you are travelling, a flask of warm water is an extra luxury. If you really want to cover all eventualities, it is possible to obtain small sterile bags of saline to flush a wound and small, sterile, antiseptic-impregnated scrubbing brushes (e.g. E-Zscrub®). There are even special spray devices for cleaning wounds, although in many situations simple thorough hosing is very effective.

Other items to consider include a **hoof pick** and decent pair of **pliers** to remove a nail or flint from a foot in an emergency. Pliers also help when a shoe is half pulled off. Easy access to the appropriate kit to remove a shoe is a good idea. Another useful tool to think about is a pair of **wire cutters** which you can lay your hands on at once in an emergency. One useful first aid gadget is a Liveryman shoemaster® which includes all these useful items in one compact, yet functional instrument.

Liveryman Shoemaster® is a useful first aid gadget. It is a multipurpose tool to make a loose or dangerous shoe safe and/or cut wire in an emergency

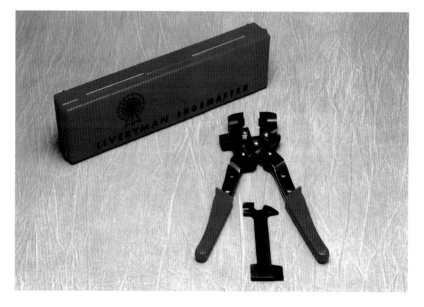

The list of possibilities to include in a first aid box is endless. I would suggest that a few strands of **bailer twine** and some **rope** are worth having. This may be invaluable in an emergency involving anything from a broken rein to a loose horse. A couple of old **towels** are worth putting on the top, as they may be useful for either pony or rider. A **notepad** and **pencil** are handy to scribble down notes in an emergency.

First aid kit contents

List of key phone numbers, e.g. vet, doctor, insurers, paper and pen
Torch, ideally a small pen torch and a larger torch (+/- spare batteries)
Thermometer
Pair of curved stainless steel scissors with blunt tips
Small pair of tweezers or forceps
Clean bucket or big bowl
Antiseptic wound cleaner, e.g. povidone-iodine (Pevidine®) or chlorhexidine
    (Hibiscrub®) and antiseptic spray
Surgical spirit
Petroleum jelly, e.g. Vaseline®
Wound gel e.g. Intrasite gel®

Dressings and bandages, including:
Cotton wool
Gamgee
Ready to use poultice, e.g. Animalintex®
Non-stick sterile dressing squares to go over wounds, e.g. Melonin®
Cotton stretch bandages, e.g. K band®
Adhesive bandages, e.g. Elastoplast®
Self-adhesive bandages, e.g. Vetrap®
Zinc oxide tape or electric insulating tape
Exercise bandages
Stable bandages

Extras
Shoe removing kit
Pliers and wire cutters
Spare hoof pick
Salt
Sterile bag of saline to flush wounds
Moist baby wipes to clean wounds
Sterile antiseptic impregnated nail brushes to clean wounds, e.g. E-Z scrub®,
manufactured by Becton Dickinson
Proprietary ice wrap, e.g. Theraflex® or cooling bandage, e.g. Bonner® bandage
Clean old towels
Bailer twine and some rope
Medications: to be discussed with your own vet and prescribed as necessary

3. WHAT TO DO WITH WOUNDS IN AN EMERGENCY

When faced with an emergency, **DO NOT PANIC!** Most accidents are not as awful as they look at first sight. If an accident does occur, always try to get help, because a problem shared is a problem halved. Try to have all the details clear in your mind so that you can describe *what* is wrong, *when* it happened and *where* you and the horse are. For a vet there is nothing worse than driving around trying to find the scene of an accident, so make sure we can find you easily. If there are enough people available, arrange for someone to stay by a phone, to relay further information and directions.

Wounds

Wounds vary from a simple cut or puncture to a major laceration. With really serious injuries, it will be obvious that immediate veterinary assistance is required. Always contact your vet if:

- any wound is bleeding profusely
- the horse is very lame, even if the wound itself is small
- any wound is more than a couple of inches long and has gone

right through the skin. If the wound gapes open, it may require stitching
- there is any suspicion of a foreign body in the wound
- there is any suspicion that a vital structure such as a joint may be involved
- the horse has *not* had an anti-tetanus vaccination.

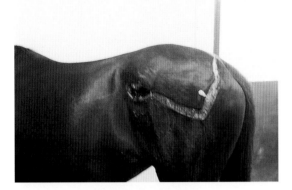

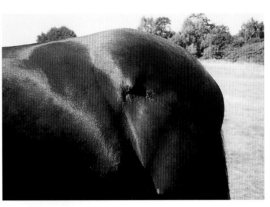

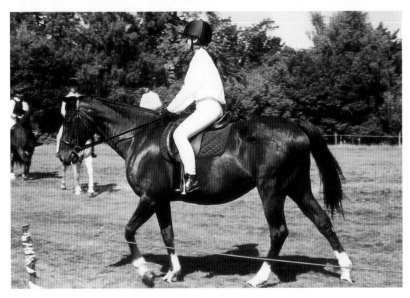

Left: This horse sustained this wound on the catch of a stable yard gate

Above: A close up of the wound when virtually healed

Bottom left: The horse which had the gate catch wound, fully healed and back in work

Remember that a wound heals from side to side, not end to end, so even if you are faced with a nasty big hole, it can heal surprisingly well. Also be aware that a little bit of blood will go a long way. Compare it to the apparently enormous flood when one pint of milk is spilt on the floor! A small amount of bleeding

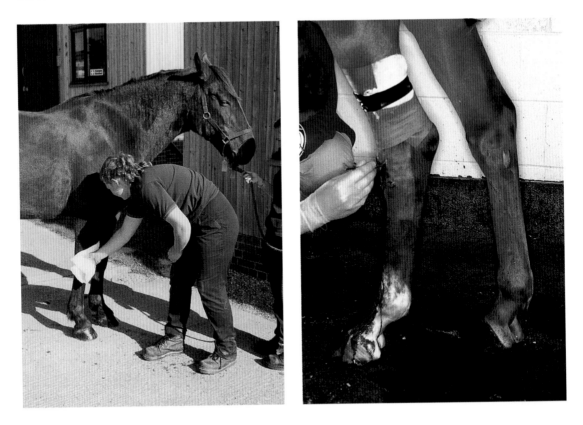

Left: Applying a pressure pad over a wound is usually more practical than a tourniquet

Right: Although rarely used, a rubber tourniquet (as shown here) can help to temporarily control bleeding

may even be beneficial as it will flush dirt and debris from a wound, but severe bleeding needs to be controlled. A Thoroughbred-size horse has to lose more than 2 gallons (9 litres) of blood before there is a serious risk of problems.

If your horse has severed an artery, this will result in the spurting of bright red blood, which can look very alarming. In such cases, try to stop the bleeding by firmly applying pressure to the wound. Make a pressure pad from a thick cloth pad, or use gamgee from your first aid kit with a non-stick dressing underneath. In an emergency, use whatever is to hand, such as a clean T-shirt, big handkerchief or towel. Press the pad against the wound and hold it there as tightly as possible. Most such wounds are on the lower limb, so a thick pressure bandage over the area will usually control bleeding. If the blood soaks through, simply put more padding over the top and apply more pressure. Cohesive elastic bandages wrapped in several moderately tight turns over a bandage pad will provide sufficient pressure to

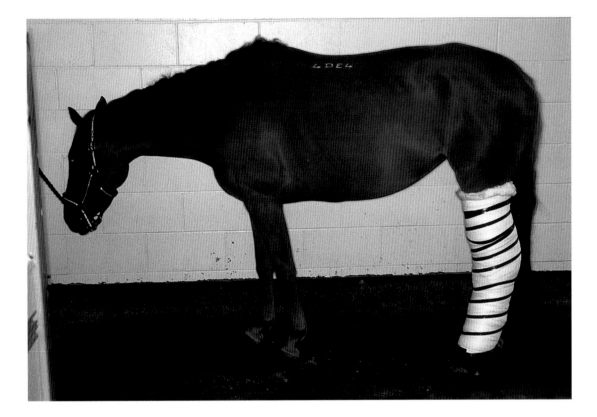

A large support bandage over a hock wound, applied with pressure to prevent the wound bleeding and to reduce bending of the limb and hence further damage to the wound

greatly reduce bleeding. This is usually better tolerated by the horse than an old-fashioned rubber or rope tourniquet and is much more practical. This is the one occasion when I would recommend applying a relatively tight bandage. Such a tight dressing should be safe for up to two hours, by which time you should have been able to contact your vet.

Talk to your horse or pony reassuringly as you keep pressure on the wound, encouraging him to stand still so that you can keep the pressure pad in place. You must keep the pressure pad in place for at least five minutes. Do not be tempted to take it off to peep underneath, as that may well restart the bleeding. Try to time the five minutes with a watch as it will seem a much longer time whilst you are doing it. Once you have got a firm comfortable pressure bandage on a wound, it is often best to leave it until help arrives.

Small wounds may have the most serious consequences. The damage caused is dependent on the wound depth, how dirty it is

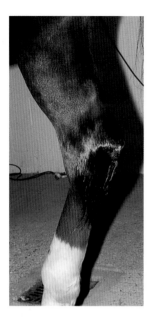

This small wound looks tiny on the outside but has penetrated vital structures within the hock, causing infection within the bone. When the horse cannot weight bear, any wound needs to be taken seriously

and whether it has involved any vital structures. Many first aid manuals warn that you should look out for so-called 'joint fluid' and that if you see an oily clear to yellow fluid discharging from a wound, then a joint must be involved. In reality, a wound is often far too dirty for you to notice this sort of discharge amongst the blood and muck already there. Also, many innocent superficial wounds will discharge clear or yellow serum which can appear frighteningly similar.

How to decide if a vital structure is involved

- Is the wound anywhere near a joint or other critical structure, such as the digital flexor tendon sheath at the back of the pastern? Remember that some joints, for instance the elbow, are very large. An injury which seems some distance away from the bending part of the joint may still communicate with it. Equally, infection can spread towards it.
- Is the horse lamer than one would expect for the size of the wound? If so, be suspicious that there is serious damage and contact your vet straightaway.

What goes wrong?

Vital structures, such as tendon sheaths and joints, are poorly designed to cope with infection. All small puncture wounds can cause complications as infection becomes trapped inside and cannot drain away. If this damage involves a joint, the infection will damage the delicate cartilage lining of the joint, producing a septic arthritis and permanent lameness unless immediate aggressive treatment is given. Similarly, infection within a tendon sheath produces inflammation and scarring which will prevent proper bending of the limb and produce permanent lameness.

Cleaning a wound may restart bleeding, so it must be done with care. Do not apply water to profusely bleeding wounds, as it will prevent clotting. If the bleeding is under control it, is safe

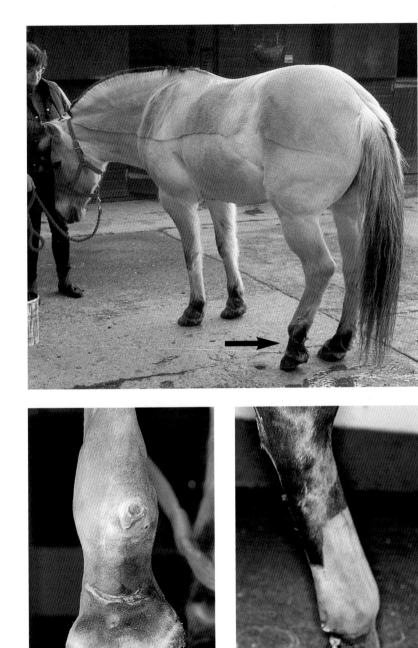

Left: This mare had a small wound at the back of the pastern, which involved the tendon sheath (arrowed). This was an emergency as she could not stand on the injured leg, and surgical treatment was required to eliminate the infection

Bottom left: A close up of a wound involving the digital sheath at the back of the pastern. This is the mare shown above at the start of surgery to clean up the injury

Bottom right: A close up of a similar wound involving the tendon sheath, showing the infected discharge, again from a tiny wound which is very painful and prevents the horse weight bearing

to clean the wound. If not, contact your vet. If you have had to apply a large pressure bandage to arrest the bleeding, leave it in place and call your vet. If a wound has bled a lot, that will clean it to some extent and cleaning it further is likely to produce more blood.

- The basic rule is **clean and cover**.
- **To clean any wound;** remove obvious dirt and grit, but do not poke around as you will introduce infection. Gentle hosing with cold water will cleanse the wound and wash away the blood. Often, underneath all the blood there will only be a tiny wound. Once this is obvious, it may help to fill the wound with a gel such as Intrasite®, which will protect it. Then, if the horse will tolerate it, trim away the hair from the edge of the wound. This allows one to see the extent of the damage and prevents hair contaminating the wound. Make sure your own hands are clean if you are touching the wound. Washing with a dilute antiseptic solution can perform further effective cleaning of the wound. (Make this solution up at the correct concentration. Do not think stronger is better as that is more liable to damage the tissues.) Alternatively, a sterile bag of saline can be used and special devices are available to attach as spray nozzles, if required.

What to put on the wound

A good rule is never put anything on a wound which you would not put in your own eye!

Most people overreact and want to apply all sorts of ointments and powders, which is not usually a good idea. The best thing is some wound gel. Most wounds occur on the lower limb, so are best dressed to protect them. Use a sterile non-adherent wound dressing such as Melonin®, to hold the wound gel in place. Then add a layer of cotton wool or gamgee, followed by a stretch bandage, e.g. K-band®, and finally something to hold it in place, e.g. insulating tape, Elastoplast® or Vetrap®. Even if you think the wound needs veterinary attention, it is a good idea to bandage it until the vet arrives. Wounds on the upper body frequently cannot be bandaged, but they should be kept as clean as possible.

Wire wounds

It is always best to unhook your horse if you can, to prevent him becoming more entangled. Wire can usually be broken by repeatedly bending it backwards and forwards in the same place, but best of all is to think ahead and choose a safe place to keep some wire cutters for when they are needed. Remember that you will have to move any other horses from the field if the fence is destroyed by a horse becoming entangled in it. Wire wounds, particularly as a result of barbed wire, are often jagged, torn lacerations which cannot easily be sutured. They will benefit from cold hosing and halting serious bleeding with pressure, just as you would with any other wounds.

Left: This horse's heel has been injured by being trapped in wire

Right: Following emergency first aid treatment it was repaired with wire, as shown

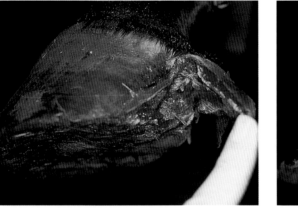

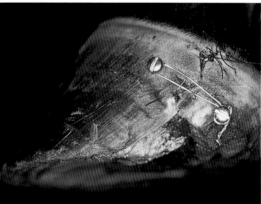

Does a wound need suturing?

If you think a wound may need to be sutured (i.e. stitched), you should consult your vet as soon as possible since a wound will heal more effectively if it is sutured whilst still fresh. This does not mean that your vet has to attend instantly as there is a six to eight hour optimum period for wound repair.

Deep punctures, very swollen or crushed wound edges, or severely contaminated or infected wounds will not be suitable for suturing, nor will wounds that are more than eight hours

A wound may need to be sutured if:
- *the edges are gaping apart*
- *it is very large or deep*
- *it is in an awkward place where it will scar.*

31

old in most cases. Your vet will be able to advise you what is best for any particular wound.

Many wounds that look appalling at first inspection will repair very well given time and proper care.

4. WHAT TO DO WITH BANDAGING IN AN EMERGENCY

Bandaging is an important part of first aid in many situations, such as:

- protecting a wound
- to control swelling
- to keep a dressing in place
- to support or protect an injury
- to restrict movement and so reduce pain.

All sorts of elegant techniques are described on how to bandage the various parts of the horse, but in any emergency the function of the bandage is far more important than its appearance. If it is being used as an emergency pressure bandage to stop bleeding until the vet arrives, and it does just that, then that it is satisfactory even if it looks a little untidy.

There is always a danger that a bandage may be put on too tight. This becomes significant if a dressing is left on for more than **two** hours, particularly if it is so tight that it becomes painful for the horse by restricting the blood supply. The horse will not always make you aware that the bandage is uncomfortable. If in doubt, always assume a bandage *is* too tight. Either get professional help to treat whatever is underneath the bandage or redo it.

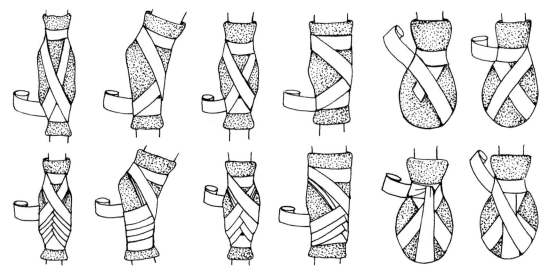

Left: How to bandage the hock making sure there is no excessive pressure on the point of the hock. Any dressing must always have padding underneath (the secondary layer)

Middle: How to bandage the knee using a figure of eight bandage, avoiding any pressure on the bony prominences at the back and sides of the knee. Again, any dressing must always have a secondary layer of padding underneath to cushion pressure

Right: How to bandage the foot

The critical points of bandaging are:

- Ensure the injured area is properly protected. If the wounds are on the horse's body it can be nearly impossible to do this properly.
- Any bandage that is applied for any reason should fit snugly but not too tightly. Avoid overtight bandaging by using plenty of padding and applying all dressings with an even tension. Remember the injured area may swell, so it is important that any dressing is well padded with cotton wool or gamgee.
- Be especially careful over prominent bony points such as the point of the hock or the back of the knee. Tight bandaging here will lead to pressure sores as there is no natural padding on the horse's limb at such points.

Any bandage is basically made up of three parts:

1 **The primary layer:** Usually this is a non-stick dressing pad, such as Melonin® or Rondopad®, which may be held in place by orthopaedic padding such as Soffban® manufactured by Smith & Nephew.
2 **The secondary layer:** This is the padding that protects the injury and controls swelling. This layer is frequently forgotten or not enough padding is used, with damaging results for the horse. With inadequate padding and overtight bandaging,

34

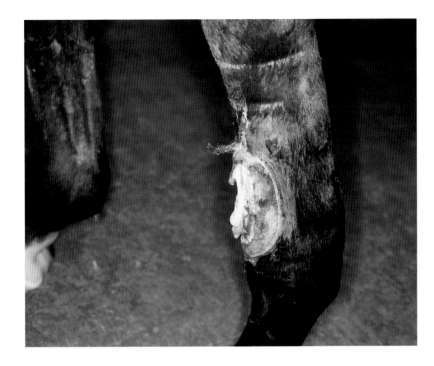

This illustrates the sort of damage that can occur if a bandage is left on too tight for too long. In this case the tendon at the front of the cannon was severely damaged. The horse made a full recovery but was left with a scar on the limb

there is a risk of causing a 'bandage bow' (i.e. localised swelling), a pressure sore or long-term scars which will leave permanent white hairs. A variety of padding materials are used. The ideal is cotton wool, as that will conform well to the shape of the leg and also tears easily. A commonly used alternative is gamgee which is also effective. The minimum amount of padding to use is once round the leg with a double layer over the tendons at the back.

3 **The tertiary layer:** This is the sealing layer which holds the dressings together and protects the layers underneath. Commonly, some sort of stretch bandage is used, that either sticks to itself, such as Vetrap®, or a stretchy conforming bandage, such as K Band®, together with adhesive tape or a sticky bandage, such as Elastoplast®. The theory is that this sealing layer should not extend beyond the edge of the underlying cotton wool or gamgee in case it causes sores by rubbing. This is particularly true with foot bandages where the heels and the back of the pastern are easily rubbed by a hard bandage. On some other areas, particularly the knee or hock, allowing a sticky bandage such as Elastoplast® to extend on to

the skin may be the only way of keeping a bandage in place. Even if this is the opposite of normal teaching, it can help as a temporary measure.

Providing a bandage is comfortable and relatively clean, there is no need to change it every day. A good bandage can be left on for up to a week. Frequently bandages are changed unnecessarily out of curiosity to check on what is underneath rather than as an essential change because the dressings are soiled. There is no need to overdo the frequency of bandage changes, especially as the bandages themselves are not cheap. Ask your vet for advice.

Left: This illustrates a method of bandaging the hock by using a zip-on lycra bandage (brown Pressage® dressing) with a proper stable bandage below to ensure it does not slip down

Right: A close-up to show the stretchy lycra Pressage® bandage, which is designed to fit the hock snugly. It is available in different sizes

Bandaging the knee and hock

Particular care is required when bandaging these areas to avoid putting excessive pressure on the prominent bones at the back and sides of the knee or point of the hock. It can be difficult to

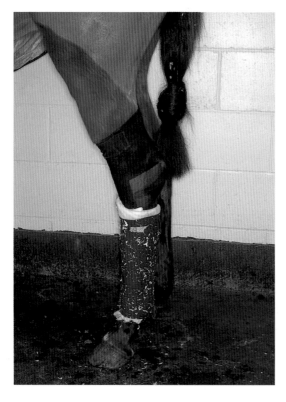

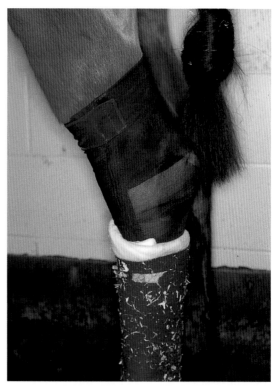

make the bandage sufficiently tight to stay on without causing injury. It helps to apply a proper stable bandage from the coronary band to the upper cannon bone to prevent the main knee or hock protector from slipping down. Another alternative is to use zip-on lycra stockings, e.g. Pressage® bandages, which work well to protect wounds on knees. They have to be removed for at least one hour in every 24 and, again, are best applied with a proper stable bandage below them to prevent any swelling below the Pressage® bandage itself. This is a far better way of holding a bandage in place rather than using sticky tape on the skin, but there are times when sticky tape on the skin is the only way of holding something in place in an emergency.

Bandaging the foot

When bandaging feet, a variety of proprietary rubber and plastic protective boots are available. The difficulty with all of these is that they tend to rub if left on when the horse is turned out. Nothing is ideal and it is best to keep a horse confined to a stable while it has a bandaged or poulticed foot. Disposable babies' nappies are a very good fit on horses' feet. Combined with sticky tape, they make an effective emergency measure. Disposable nappies are ideal for keeping a poultice in place when a horse has pus in the foot. Aluminium foil can be inserted as an insulating layer beneath a warm poultice to help keep the heat in. Commercial poultice bandages, e.g. Animalintex®, are very useful, particularly for pus in the foot (see below).

How to apply a foot poultice

The aim is to apply the warm poultice to the sore area of the foot, e.g. when a horse has a foot abscess. Traditionally, this is said to help draw out infection and stimulate the circulation to the injured area. In reality, its main role is to soften hard hooves so that it is easier to pare the sole to expose and drain an abscess. Poulticing the foot for more than three days can, in fact, be damaging as the excess moisture will damage the hoof wall and make

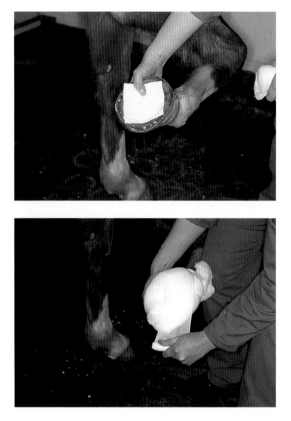

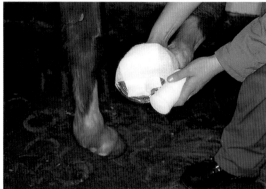

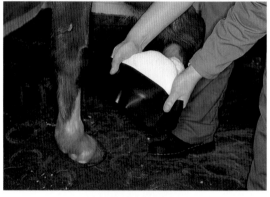

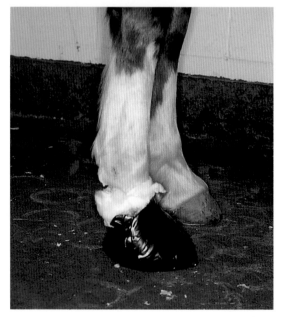

How to fit a foot poultice

Top left: The hot piece of poultice (in this case, Animalintex®) is applied to the sole of the foot

Top right: A layer of padding is applied to the foot over the poultice and then held in place with a conforming bandage

Above: The bandage is criss-crossed over the foot

Above right: Securing the padding and poultice with 10 cm black sticky tape

Right: The poulticed foot

it more difficult to refit a shoe. Poulticing any area for more than three days may actually delay healing.

If you are applying a poultice as a short-term remedy, exactly how it is done is not critical just as long as you manage to apply the poultice to the right area and keep it safely in place. It is rather like wrapping up a Christmas present. There are many ways of doing that and just as many ways of poulticing the foot.

You will require:

- a poultice, e.g. the medicated commercially available poultice Animalintex® is a good first choice
- a square of gamgee, cotton wool or a nappy as padding
- a square of aluminium foil
- a conforming bandage
- 7.5 cm or 10 cm black sticky tape, plastic bags or a poultice boot
- hot water
- gamgee and a stable bandage which should be applied to the limb as a normal support bandage as well as the foot poultice.

It is important to:

- smear some petroleum jelly (e.g. Vaseline®) on the heels first to protect them
- ensure the poultice is not so hot that it will burn the horse. If it is only to be applied to the sole and is definitely not in contact with the skin, then it can be hotter, otherwise check it against your own skin before applying it to the horse
- keep the horse in once it is poulticed to prevent the poultice falling off.

The hot poultice should be applied to the area of concern, e.g. the sole of the foot. If you are using Animalintex® cut a piece to the right size to cover the area you need and immerse it in hot water. The excess water is then squeezed out and the poultice applied. The plastic backing layer is meant to be on the side furthermost away from the foot itself. Ideally, a layer of aluminium foil should be put on top of that to help keep the heat in and

A heel which has been rubbed and burnt as a consequence of too hot a poultice being applied to the skin. The bandages which had been applied to the heel had also rubbed and exacerbated the problem

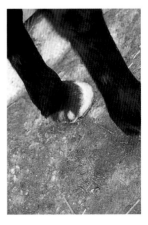

then a layer of padding, such as cotton wool or gamgee, should be used. A bandage is then wrapped around the foot in the same way as any foot bandage, or a disposable nappy can be used to hold everything in place. For extra padding, use more than one nappy. Secure the padding with either 7.5 cm or 10 cm black sticky tape, i.e. duct tape. If you want to protect the foot thoroughly (and make it sweat) use a plastic bag as well. To allow more breathing, use more gamgee and no nappies and a conforming bandage rather than plastic tape. Traditionally, people used to protect the foot with a piece of hessian sacking, but these days an old sock might be more easily available or you could use a proprietary boot, designed to keep a poultice in place. Instead of using Animalintex®, it is possible to use a bran poultice, i.e. packing the foot with moist bran, sometimes mixed with Epsom salts in the proportions of roughly one part Epsom salts to two parts of bran. This is messy, but can be bandaged against the foot with the help of plastic bags, sacking or nappies. Any poultice should be changed once daily or sometimes twice daily. Never continue poulticing for more than three days without consulting your vet.

A full limb bandage or splint

If a horse has a badly injured limb, such as a broken bone (i.e. fracture) on the lower limb, or damage to the joint or tendon, it may require a proper splint. The aim of a splint is to:

- prevent further injury
- stabilise the limb
- prevent infection of any open wound
- make the horse comfortable to travel.

It is recognised that the initial first aid treatment of any fracture is a major factor in the eventual recovery of the horse. If an injured horse is going to have to be transported to an equine hospital for diagnosis and treatment, it is vital that his injuries are properly stabilised before he is moved. Your veterinary surgeon will need to decide how to fit such a dressing since different

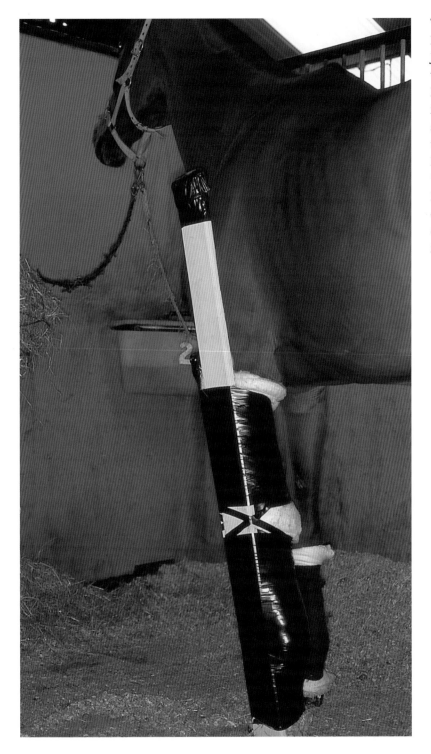

This horse has a full limb bandage (Robert Jones type dressing with a splint) on the left limb to support a fracture. There is also a support bandage on the opposite limb. Note that the horse is 'cross-tied' with two lead ropes so that he cannot lie down and damage the limb further

Right: This horse has a
full limb bandage for
travel including two
wooden splints to help
support the injury

Below: A commercially
available splint, which a
vet may use to support
a lower limb injury in
an emergency

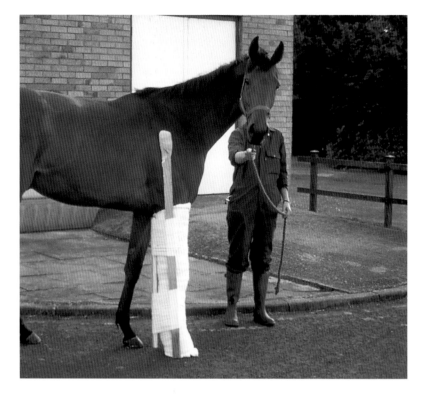

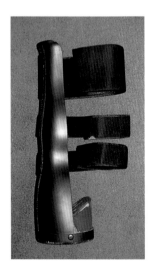

splinting techniques will be needed depending on the area of
damage. Ideally, a splint should immobilise the joints above and
below the area of damage, where this is possible. Once the limb
has been splinted appropriately, the horse will usually feel more
confident and will calm down, which further emphasises the
importance of rapid first aid support.

Occasionally a vet may fit a ready-made splint, e.g. the Kimzey
splint or monkey splint, which provides effective first aid support to an injury such as a suspected fracture of the lower limb.
More commonly, an enormous padded bandage, known as a
Robert Jones dressing, will be applied by your vet to support the
injured leg. Many first aid guides imply that this is something you
can apply yourself. However, unless you are confident that you
know what you are doing, it is better to seek immediate help
from your vet. A badly or inappropriately applied splint can make
an injury worse by causing further destabilisation. Also, it is
unlikely that you will have enough dressings available to do a
proper job. Furthermore, your vet is likely to want to take the

dressing off as soon as he or she arrives in order to assess the damage thoroughly.

Bandaging other areas

It can be extremely difficult to bandage the upper limbs, head or body of a horse. If any bandage is used, either the horse must be supervised or you must be one hundred per cent confident that the bandage will not slip and frighten the animal. This is particularly true of any dressing that is put on the head, as any horse will panic if his vision is obscured. For this reason any dressing on the head must be applied very carefully, if at all. Bandages on the head are rarely necessary, however, as head wounds heal very well in most cases. When a dressing on the head is needed, the stretchy nylon protective hoods worn to keep horses clean may help keep a bandage in place. Another option, particularly when trying to protect the horse's eye, especially from self-inflicted injury, is to use a traditional racing hood with blinkers.

Bandaging the upper hind limb is almost impossible, and the top of the forearm is nearly as difficult as no dressing will stay in place. With the foreleg the only way is also to bandage the whole lower limb beneath the area in question so the dressing cannot slip down. With a back leg, it is usually far safer to leave the area

The minimum amount of material needed to construct a Robert Jones bandage for a full limb is:
- *8 to 10 rolls of cotton wool*
- *15 to 20 rolls of conforming bandage*
- *6 to 7 rolls of elastic adhesive tape*
i.e. more than is available in the standard stable first aid kit. If it is to be done properly you will need your vet for this first aid unless you have previous training and experience.

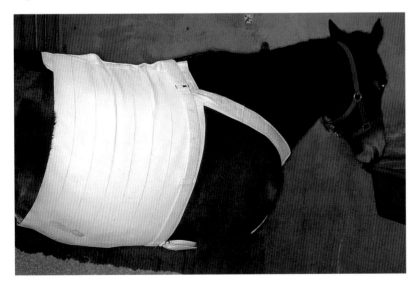

A purpose-made belly bandage fitted to a horse following colic surgery

unbandaged and concentrate your efforts on keeping the injury clean instead.

Whole body bandages are rarely necessary or effective. Occasionally a clean sheet or something similar may be used as immediate first aid to protect a wound. Vets often use purpose-designed belly wraps, particularly after colic surgery, to help support an abdominal incision. These can sometimes be used to help support other abdominal wounds.

Protecting the bandage

Some horses will develop a habit of tearing or chewing at their dressings or bandages. In a few cases this is just bad behaviour, but in most it is an indication that the horse is uncomfortable. You should seek your vet's advice to ensure there is no underlying reason for bandage ripping. If you have established that it is a habit that needs to be prevented, then you can try a variety of alternatives. Anti-chewing pastes are available, or you can use something, such as hot English mustard, which can be applied to an old bandage or stocking over the outer dressing. These are messy and do not always work.

A better alternative is to try an anti-rug-chewing bib or seek your vet's assistance to fit a 'cradle'. This is a device fitted around the neck, made from pieces of wood (like ladder rungs) separat-

A cradle

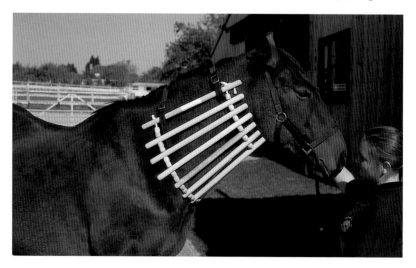

ed by rope, webbing or leather. Such a device can prevent a horse bending his neck to reach limb bandages. Another less kind alternative, but which may be the only option in some cases, is to keep the horse tied up. If you are unsure on how to manage this problem, ask your vet.

Travelling bandages

On the basis that prevention is better than cure, good protective travelling gear can help avoid injuries whilst travelling. Proper protective bandages should be applied to all four limbs when a horse travels. Any protection is better than nothing, but good bandages should not slip up or down, as well as providing adequate protection for the knees and hocks if the horse should fall whilst travelling. A poll guard is a sensible precaution too, since a blow to the head, caused if a horse rears up or falls over backwards, can be fatal.

Left: This poll guard will help to protect a horse whilst travelling as a blow to the head if a horse rears up or falls over backwards, can be fatal

Right: Poll guard

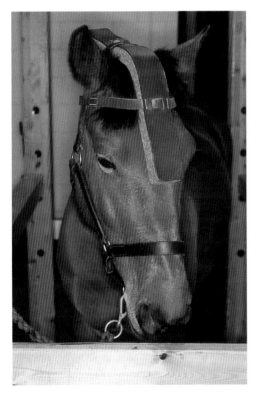

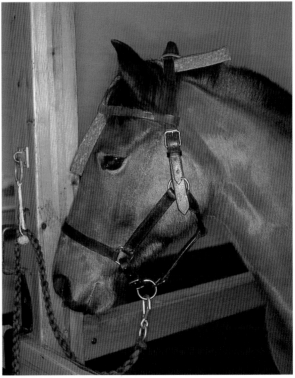

5. WHAT TO DO WHEN FACED WITH SOME OF THE MORE COMMON EMERGENCIES

It is impossible to describe every situation or provide set rules for when to call your vet, but common concerns are covered below.

Azoturia

Azoturia is also known as 'set-fast', 'tying-up' or, most properly, equine rhabdomyolysis syndrome (ERS). It is a disturbance of muscle function, similar to muscle cramp, which can occur when out riding or just after exercise. It can be very distressing to both horse and rider.

What to look for

The horse seems unwilling to go, he may take short steps and feel very unsteady or stiff in his back legs. The muscles of the hindquarters feel hot and hard. In some very rare, severe cases the horse seizes up and cannot move. The horse may even collapse and be unable to stand. The signs can be confused with those of colic. The horse may appear very distressed and uncomfortable. Basically, the muscles hurt and this alarms the horse. He will have a raised pulse and a slight increase in temperature. There may be frequent attempts to urinate but muscle pain may prevent him standing in the normal stance to stale. With severe muscle damage, the urine may be a red-brown to dark chocolate colour. The whole condition will always seem much worse in a nervous animal which tends to panic. A nervous pony may be much more distressed than a stoical hunter, despite a similar level of stiffness.

What to do

- If you had a bad cramp, you would not want to move either, so in these circumstances you must stop and let the horse rest.
- Put rugs or coats over the horse's back to keep him warm.
- Try to encourage the horse to drink, which is obviously not always possible. Fluids will help flush out the kidneys and reduce the problems associated with muscle breakdown. At the same time, it is sensible to watch that the horse is urinating properly. Hay and a wet bran mash should be offered as a fluid-containing feed. Bran is not an ideal *regular* feed to recommend for these cases, but is useful following an attack. The very fact of giving the horse a haynet and feed may help to reduce its anxiety.
- If at or near to home, the horse should be put in a stable and offered water. A thick dry bed should be provided in case the horse wants to lie down. If he does go down, let him lie down and do not force him to stand up again.
- If away from home, attempt to obtain help to get you home. Try to arrange transport for the horse rather than riding back to base. A lorry is best as it calls for less muscular work for a horse to stand in, compared to a trailer where the horse has to brace himself more using his already sore muscles.
- In the worst and very rare cases, when the horse cannot move and may not be able to stand, contact your vet immediately requesting emergency attention. Milder cases may be managed by rugging or warming the back and hindquarters, but you should still consult your vet for advice.

47

How to make a
bran mash:
1 kg bran
30 g salt
300 ml molasses
2 litres hot water
Stir thoroughly.
Leave to stand for
10 minutes before
feeding.

Once a horse has had an episode of azoturia, you should discuss future management with your vet. Blood tests may be necessary to monitor progress. Whilst the horse is recovering, he should be kept either in a stable or a small paddock and fed on a low energy diet. It is best not to return to work until you have the all clear from the vet.

Azoturia is a condition where it makes sense to minimise the distance the horse has to travel, so ask the vet to come to you rather than take the horse to the vet. If it happens at a competition, ideally the vet may be able to treat the horse at the place of occurrence. If possible, it is best to avoid moving the horse a long distance either under his own steam or in a horsebox.

Breathing problems

Breathing problems can cause a horse to suffer the equivalent of an asthmatic attack with signs of respiratory distress, e.g. laboured breathing ('heaves'), flaring nostrils and sometimes sweating or coughing.

In the UK, most cases are associated with a dust allergy, but are occasionally due to other conditions such as pneumonia. In a similar way to people with asthma, who are allergic to certain things which make them breathless and wheezy, horses develop **chronic obstructive pulmonary disease (COPD)**. COPD is also known as **chronic small airway disease (SAD)** and **chronic pulmonary disease (CPD)**, **broken wind**, **heaves** or **stable cough**. In the worst cases, an affected horse will be perpetually breathless and/or coughing. In mild cases they may just cough occasionally and have less stamina. The disease develops as a result of an allergic response to organic dusts, particularly hay and straw dust and the fungal spores that they contain. Occasionally horses will be allergic to pollens. If a sensitised horse is exposed to a large amount of the allergen that affects him, he will become ill. This is the commonest reason for breathing difficulties in horses in the UK.

Overall breathing difficulties can be due either to problems for the lungs in taking on board enough oxygen or to an obstruction somewhere in the airways which prevents the air getting in or out of the lungs.

48

If the lungs are involved the horse may be wheezing, coughing or breathing rapidly and sometimes may have a sticky white/yellow discharge from the nose. If there is a blockage somewhere in the airway, then the horse may make a loud respiratory noise, i.e. it will sound as if he is roaring or snoring.

Immediate action

If the horse is gasping and really breathless and this does not improve within an hour, contact your vet straightaway, particularly if the condition has come on rapidly.

The horse should be placed in a dust-free open airy space, e.g. a paddock, and kept quiet and under close observation. Obviously, any exercise is liable to make breathlessness worse, so do not make the animal move unnecessarily.

Check the horse's temperature to see if he has a fever. This is unlikely but if he has, this suggests an infection and you should contact your vet straightaway.

- If there is severe coughing which will not stop, again it is sensible to contact your vet straightaway as the horse may have something stuck in his airways or gullet.
- If the horse has recently suffered an injury to the chest, again contact your vet straightaway.
- If there is a new loud snoring/roaring sound all the time, contact your vet straightaway. If this noise is only present at exercise, it is not so urgent, but you should still talk to your vet within the week if it does not go away.

What your vet will do

This depends on the suspected cause. Drugs can be prescribed which will rapidly help many breathing problems, although they may only control the signs temporarily rather than provide a cure. In some cases your vet may recommend inserting an endoscope, which will allow him or her to examine the inside of the nose, throat, windpipe and lungs, to find out what is wrong.

Cast horses

A **cast horse** is one that has rolled against a wall in the stable, become wedged there and cannot get up. More than one person is needed to right a large horse. The ideal is to have lunge lines or long ropes and loop these over the foot on the limb nearest the wall just above or below the fetlock. Occasionally simply pulling the forelimbs round will enable a horse to right himself. Usually both back and front legs have to be pulled over to move the horse away from the wall. Stand well back and allow the horse to get up on his own, then, whilst reassuring the horse, carefully remove the ropes. It is most important to keep yourself from being injured. Once the horse is up, check him carefully for injuries. Call the vet straightaway if there are major injuries.

- If a horse becomes cast regularly, he may do better if kept in a larger stable and/or wears an anti-cast roller. Also, a deeper bed with big banks may prevent him from becoming wedged against the wall.
- A horse may become cast as a result of rolling because he has had a touch of colic, so watch him carefully once he is back on his feet.

Horses cast in a ditch or bog

Professional and strong help is usually required to free a horse in this situation. If in a ditch, it is important to roll the horse right way up, so he can then stand on his own. If in a bog, a horse should not be pulled out forwards, as this will tend to drive his front legs in deeper. Your vet will advise on the appropriate attachment of ropes (around the chest behind the withers, ideally with broad straps or a sling) to pull a horse out spine (i.e. back) first. Remember that this is potentially dangerous as a horse can suddenly struggle free so it is essential to avoid human injury by keeping out of harm's way. A horse struggling to right himself will trample on someone in his panic. Horses can behave unpredictably and are potentially dangerous, so take all possible care to avoid injury. In some cases your vet may administer a tranquilliser to enable the horse to be manipulated into a safe position.

Choke

Choke occurs when a horse gets food stuck in his oesophagus (gullet). The results can appear dramatic. One moment the horse is fine and the next he is coughing and spluttering with saliva and food drooling from mouth and nostrils. It is usually less serious than it seems and the majority of cases will clear themselves rapidly with no treatment.

- First aid treatment is to prevent the horse from eating or drinking anything further. It is best to put him in a box with no hay or water and non-edible bedding, then contact your vet for advice. By the time you have done so, the obstruction will frequently have cleared.

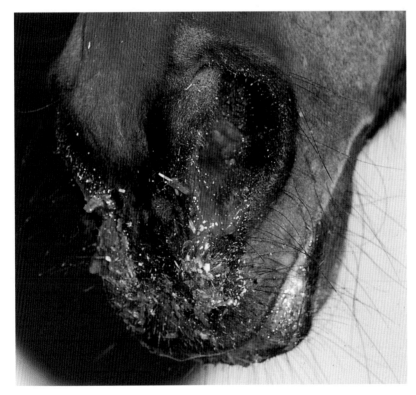

A horse with choke will have food and saliva draining from his nostrils and sometimes from the mouth as well

51

- Occasionally a lump of food can be felt on the left side of the neck. Massaging this gently may help it to disperse.
- Keep the horse quiet, with his head low to allow saliva to drain.
- If the obstruction does not shift within a few hours, you will need help from your vet.

What your vet will do

This depends on how long the choke has been going on and how uncomfortable the horse is. The majority of cases will need very little treatment apart from injections to relax the muscles and allow the obstruction to pass. If the problem persists, the vet may use more aggressive treatments to move the blockage. Sometimes a stomach tube is passed down the oesophagus and fluid gently pumped through to soften and shift the blockage. Giving the horse large amounts of fluids as an intravenous drip will help, as he can become dehydrated through continually dribbling saliva and being unable to drink because of the blockage. On rare occasions a general anaesthetic is needed so that the blockage can be dislodged using various surgical procedures.

What you should do afterwards

Immediately after an obstruction has cleared, offer only water for twelve hours and then only soft food and water for the next twelve hours, because of pain in the gullet and the increased chance of a repeat obstruction. Many horses develop choke because they are greedy eaters that bolt their food. If this is the case, it is important to slow down their eating, e.g. by putting a large round stone or salt lick in their manger so they have to nibble around it, and using a hay net with small holes so it takes longer for them to eat.

Classically, horses are said to choke on unsoaked sugar beet. If this feed is used, it must be well soaked before it is given to any horse (follow the manufacturer's instructions). Also, the supply of unsoaked sugar beet must be kept somewhere safe where it cannot be accessed by any hungry horses or ponies.

Colic

The word 'colic' means abdominal pain. Signs include:

- restlessness
- turning and looking at the flank
- kicking at the abdomen
- sweating
- rolling
- digging up the bed
- lying down for longer than normal
- repeated stretching as if to urinate
- dropping suddenly to the floor and then rolling violently
- crouching as if wanting to lie down, i.e. buckling at the knees
- failure to pass any droppings in a 24-hour period.

In severe cases of colic, the affected horse can thrash around alarmingly due to the pain. If the horse is violent, do not risk being injured. If you can, try to calm the distressed animal; getting him up and walking him, particularly on hard ground where he will not want to roll, may help. If he is determined to go down, make sure he is in a big enough box where he will not easily get cast or, if practical, put him in a sand school or field where

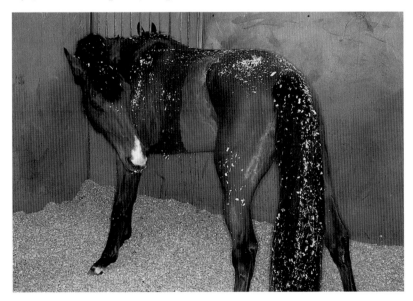

A horse showing colic pain will turn to look at his flank and may often be covered in shavings from rolling, as shown

A post-mortem picture
of a twisted gut from a
case of severe colic.
Surgery would have
been the only way to
correct this

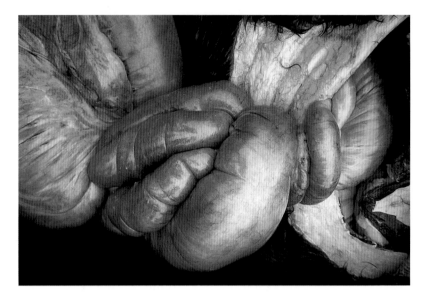

he is less likely to damage himself. It is a myth that a colicking
horse will twist his bowel by rolling. If a violently colicking horse
is rolling, it is probably because he has already tangled up his
intestines and rolling is his instinctive way of trying to sort this
out. It is unlikely to help, but provided he does not injure himself
by doing it, rolling as such will not make a bad situation any
worse.

- Colic is the classic case where delay can be dangerous. No
  matter how experienced you are, if even a mild colic persists
  for more than half an hour, or a colic subsides but then recurs,
  you should at least speak to your vet. If there is any doubt,
  arrange for the horse to be checked by your vet. If the colic
  appears to have cleared on its own, still ensure someone
  checks the horse two to four hours later to make sure there is
  no recurrence. Every year we see many horses with severe
  colic, which have been in agony all night. Controlling colic is
  a very good argument for a regular late-night check of your
  horse. If a horse is left unattended for twelve hours or more,
  an initially mild colic in the evening may have progressed to a
  more serious condition when found the following morning.
- If there is any possibility that a horse may need surgery for
  colic, it should be travelled to the appropriate equine hospital

before its condition deteriorates. It is far better that it is travelled unnecessarily rather than waiting till it is too ill to make any journey (except to heaven!).

• Colic drenches are unlikely to help and should not be given without contacting your vet first. Occasionally your vet may recommend a drench with a small amount of a spirit such as

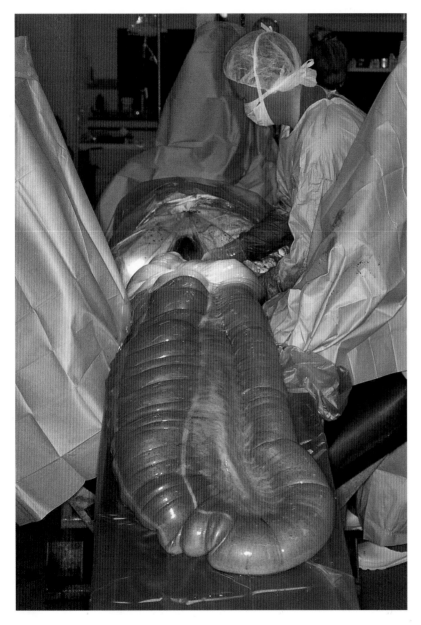

A horse under general anaesthesia undergoing surgery for colic. The colon (large bowel) is visible outside the horse's abdomen on the operating table

55

brandy (say a teacupful for a Thoroughbred-size horse). This may be effective in controlling mild pain without the danger of disguising a serious abdominal catastrophe.

- If a horse is trying to roll, it may help to walk the horse for up to 30 minutes. It is wrong to continually walk a horse with colic for hours. If he does not rapidly improve, you should seek immediate veterinary advice.

Whilst you are waiting for the vet to arrive, remove all feed from the horse's reach, but leave water available. Have water, soap and towel ready for the vet, as he or she is likely to need it. If the colic is severe, the horse may need to be transported to an equine clinic for further treatment, so make sure you have transport available and are ready to go.

The critical thing with any colic is catching it early. Hopefully, horses are checked on frequently, so any signs of colic are detected straightaway. Colic is more successfully managed if treatment is started at once. Painkillers work better if they are given before the pain takes hold. In the five to ten per cent of cases that require surgery, the chances of success are much greater if an operation is carried out as soon as possible.

What the vet will do for colic

Every time a vet examines a horse with colic he or she has to decide whether it is a surgical or medical case. The majority are the latter and respond well to pain-killing drugs. Sometimes the passage of a stomach tube relieves pressure in the stomach and allows administration of large volumes of liquid paraffin or other substances. The vet often performs a rectal or internal examination to help diagnose the cause of the colic. The vet may also take a sample of fluid from inside the abdomen. This is know as a belly tap or peritoneal tap. By looking at the fluid, your vet will have another clue as to what is wrong and if surgery is required. The few cases that require surgery may temporarily appear to improve with painkillers, but will deteriorate and die without emergency surgical repair. It can be very hard to distinguish whether or not surgery is necessary. Surgery can be life saving. If

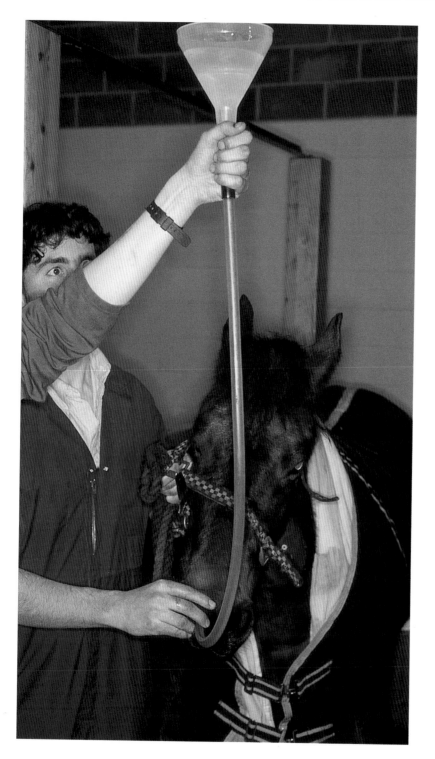

A stomach tube being passed and liquid paraffin being administered to a case of colic

the bowel is twisted or completely obstructed, drugs, drenches or walking the horse will not produce a cure.

Many horses have undergone successful colic surgery and returned to full work. It is best to be ready for a crisis before it occurs. Think now whether it would be right to submit your horse to costly surgery. Insurance is well worth having to cover this eventuality. It is better to know that your horse can have the veterinary care he needs rather than what you can afford.

Collapse

If a serious accident happens and your horse is down on the ground and cannot get up, do not try to move him. Be careful to approach from behind his back to avoid being kicked if he tries to stand. Try to encourage the horse to stand, but be ready to move quickly out of the way yourself. If out riding, undo the girths if you can do so without risk to yourself.

- If a horse is unable to stand there is likely to be something seriously wrong, so call your vet immediately.

How to assist a horse to stand

It is impossible to lift a large horse to his feet using manpower. You can only guide his own efforts. A horse that has fallen on a slippery surface should be manoeuvred so that any slope can be used to his advantage; i.e. the horse should be facing either downhill or uphill. The front feet should be pulled out forwards and placed on a non-slip surface, e.g. rubber car mats. The hindlimbs need to be under the body and not stuck out backwards. Usually two people should assist, with one holding a leadrope attached to a headcollar and the other the tail. All human effort should be reserved for when the horse makes his big effort. A certain amount of persuasion may be needed. It is vital to ensure that nobody is hurt, so follow instructions and be ready for the horse to move suddenly: expect the unexpected!

Whilst waiting for the vet, put a coat or sweater under the horse's head to protect the eye nearest the ground from injury. If a horse is struggling to rise but cannot do so, kneel high on the neck pressing his head on the ground to prevent further struggling or, even better if you feel capable, keep a knee on the neck and raise the horse's nose when it attempts to struggle. Always sit on the mane side of the neck; if you are on the other side, you are too close to the front legs and may be kicked as the horse tries to stand. Anything like this is potentially dangerous. It is most important to ensure you are not injured as this will obviously not help your horse. Covering the upper eye will help to keep a frightened horse quiet. Always talk soothingly to calm him and yourself. Remember that a horse that has fallen down may just be winded and, given time and help, he may well be fine.

Diarrhoea

Diarrhoea in a foal justifies contacting your vet the same day. If an adult horse with diarrhoea is bright, well, eating and drinking, it is unlikely to be an immediate emergency, but your vet should be rung if it continues for more than 48 hours. If an adult horse with diarrhoea is ill, particularly if he shows signs of colic or has a raised temperature, consult your vet straightaway. First aid for an adult horse with diarrhoea should include:

- stabling the horse
- feeding good hay, but no grass and allowing plenty of water
- checking your worming regime
- there is always a remote risk that diarrhoea can spread to other horses or people. For this reason it is sensible to be particularly careful with hygiene yourself and keep the affected horse in, away from other horses
- cleaning the dock area and buttocks. Applying petroleum jelly (Vaseline®) can reduce skin damage
- it may be necessary to bandage the tail to keep it clean.

A horse with a painful eye will tend to keep the eye closed, especially in bright light. The eye will weep excessively

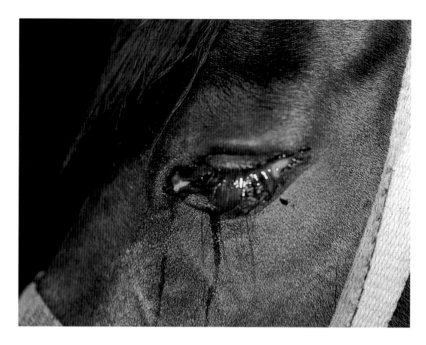

Eye injuries and disease

Eye injuries and diseases are potentially serious. Apart from the obvious wounds to eyelids, damage to the eye may also be indicated by a weepy eye and attempts to keep the affected eye shut, especially in bright light. If your horse is keeping his eye partially or completely closed, it means it hurts. There may be something in his eye. Infections or foreign bodies in the eye cause reddening of the membranes around the eye and an obvious dirty discharge from the eye itself.

Prompt treatment is particularly important with eye problems. You should always consult your veterinary surgeon rather than try some eye ointment you might have available, which may be totally inappropriate for the condition in question.

A severe eye injury or an obviously painful eye will require attention as soon as possible from your vet, but for the majority of eye problems you should, at the very least, discuss the problem with your vet the day the injury occurs. A non-painful slightly runny eye or a swelling adjacent to the eye is unlikely to be a critical emergency, but if there is any cause for concern regarding an eye condition, talk to your vet rather than leave it. A painful eye should never be ignored. It is not worth taking risks with eyes, as they are irreplaceable and matters can deteriorate so rapidly.

- First aid for eyes includes never trying to force the eyelids open if the eye is shut. This can damage the eye further. It is far better to allow your vet to do it using appropriate painkillers to help the horse.
- If there is something sticking out of the eyeball, never pull it out, as it may be a part of the inside of the eye itself that is plugging a wound that has perforated the front of the eye. Gently bathe any foreign bodies that surround the eye if you can do so without causing discomfort. The best eyewash is sterile saline (small bags can be bought specifically for this purpose), or a proper medical artificial tears solution. Boiled and cooled water is a good alternative in an emergency. If in doubt, consult your vet before using anything in the eye which may irritate it further.

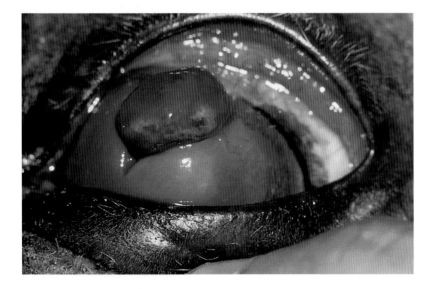

This horse has sustained a serious cut to the front of the eye. This is a good example why something that appears to be sticking into the eye should not be pulled out as here it is actually part of the eye itself

- The irritation and discomfort from an eye problem will often tempt a horse to rub his eye, which will inevitably make things worse. Any sensible way of preventing this happening is a very useful first aid measure. One of the best

61

ways of preventing a horse rubbing his eye is to use a pair of blinkers to protect the eye. In an emergency you could stay with a horse to prevent him rubbing whilst professional help is sought. If the horse is well behaved, an ice pack (frozen peas would do!) in between layers of soft clean cloth held against the eye for five minutes may help to soothe it.

- Many horses with eye problems are sensitive to light. They may feel better if placed in a quiet, dust-free, fly-free, dark stable.
- It will also help if you wipe away the discharge from a runny eye as the discharge will attract flies and exacerbate the problem. Application of petroleum jelly (Vaseline®) to the face around the eye may reduce scalding of the skin.
- Feeding hay on the floor will help to stop falling dust irritating an already sore eye.

The same basic approach applies whatever the actual eye problem.

A pony with a sore eye will often try to rub it. This can be prevented by the use of blinkers, as shown

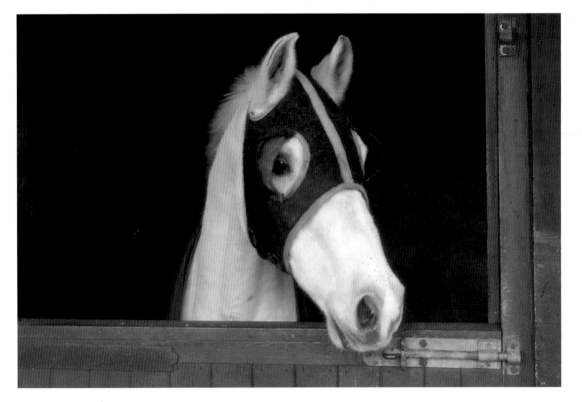

Common eye conditions

Normally there is a 'clear window' at the front of the eye, known as the cornea. As the horse's eyes are so large and stick out on either side of the head, it is the cornea which is prone to damage. Damage to the cornea can be very painful and may be obvious but pain within the eye is often as bad.

A CLOUDY EYE

When the clear cornea is damaged, it becomes cloudy or foggy (known properly as corneal oedema) and the horse can no longer see through it. This can occur for a variety of reasons. The most critical is a condition known as a **melting ulcer**. This is a genuine emergency because of the speed with which the cornea can perforate. The cornea does not have a blood supply, so bacteria can flourish in and around any injury to it. Some particularly vicious bacteria produce enzymes that dissolve the cells of the cornea, turning it to a jelly-like liquid. The integrity of the cornea can be threatened within a few hours. If it does perforate, the eye is almost certainly lost, so early and aggressive treatment is essential.

CORNEAL ULCERS

More common are ordinary **corneal ulcers**, which are sometimes seen as a white spot on the eye. Most ulcers do not develop into the melting type, but should still be seen by a vet in order to start

Left: A melting ulcer, where the eye appears to dissolve, is a genuine emergency. In this case, you can see that the membranes around the eye (the conjunctiva) are also red and painful

Right: The horse has an ulcer in the eye (arrowed). The blood vessels growing across the eye are nature's attempt to heal it

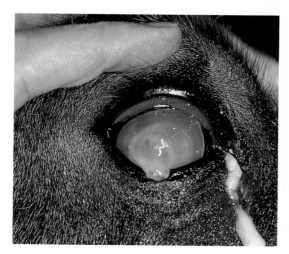

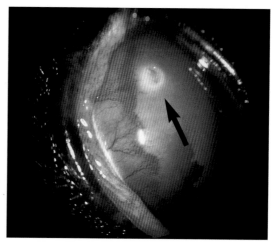

treatment as soon as possible. The chance of a rapid recovery is increased the sooner treatment is started. The maximum thickness of the cornea is approximately 1 mm, therefore a superficial ulcer can rapidly become a perforated ulcer. A veterinary examination will rule out other serious eye conditions such as melting ulcers, foreign bodies and other damage within the eye itself.

A RED EYE

It is important to try and establish which bit of the eye is red to understand what is wrong. If the membranes around the eye are red and swollen, then it is likely that the horse is suffering from conjunctivitis, sometimes called '**pink eye**'. This is very common and has a variety of causes. It can be due to an irritant such as a piece of bedding getting into the eye. It can also be caused by eye infections which are frequently spread from horse to horse by flies. Occasionally it is an indication of a whole body infection such the viral infection of **equine viral arteritis**. Bathing the eye may help, along with keeping the flies away, but if it does not improve rapidly you should contact your vet.

Occasionally the membranes surrounding the eye can become very irritated and swell up so much that they can barely be seen. This is rare but can occur as a result of a severe irritant, particularly if a chemical has splashed into the eyes or there has been some kind of allergic reaction. This is very sore and the eye will usually weep profusely as well. Most will settle down if the irritant is removed. You should ring your vet straightaway and it may help to bathe the eye gently whilst they are on their way to see you. If the eye has definitely been splashed by a chemical or there is a known allergen, e.g. pollen, in the eye, then this is a case where it is justified in washing the eye with copious amounts of tap water. If you do use water, ensure it is as clean as possible.

Sometimes the eyeball itself will look red. This may be because it is filled with blood, sometimes as a result of trauma. It may also be due to inflammation within the eye, associated with internal problems such as **moon blindness** or **equine periodic ophthalmia** (see below). In these cases the eye will be painful and you should get assistance from your vet immediately.

A RUNNY EYE

There are several reasons why tears will overflow from the eye. These include an excess of tear production, a reduction of the ability of the tear duct to drain the tears and loss of the close-fitting nature of the eyelids. If too much tear fluid is being produced it indicates that the eye is irritated and inflamed. The natural response is to produce fluid to wash whatever is wrong away. Many horses have slightly watery eyes occasionally without significant problems. The time to worry is if:

- it appears painful
- the eye is held closed
- the discharge persists or becomes infected, i.e. goes yellowy pus coloured.

If this is the case you should contact your vet for an appointment.

AN EYELID WOUND

You should ask your vet to examine and repair any eyelid wound involving the eyelid margin to avoid complications later. If repaired properly such wounds usually heal very well. If left to heal on their own, you can get serious scarring and damage to the eye itself.

MOON BLINDNESS

This is properly called **equine recurrent uveitis (ERU)**. This and other causes of inflammation in the front part of the eyeball (properly called **uveitis**) should be considered, as this is a significant cause of blindness in the horse. Unfortunately many cases are not detected in the early stages when they have the best chance of responding to treatment. Signs to watch for are:

- pain: a watery eye, a closed eye and avoidance of bright light
- reduced ability to see
- reduction in the size of the pupil if you can see it.

The only way of controlling this is early, aggressive and frequent treatment.

First aid is of limited benefit. It is far better to call your vet at the

This horse is suffering from moon blindness (equine recurrent uveitis). The eye has a watery discharge and the pupil is constricted. The surface of the eye (the cornea) looks cloudy and the membranes around the eye are red, i.e. there is conjunctivitis

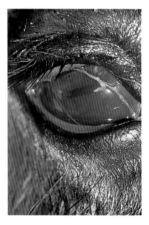

first suspicion of the complaint. Unfortunately it is a condition that tends to recur. If you have a horse that is known to have this, it may be worth discussing with your vet the option of having some appropriate anti-inflammatory drugs in your first aid kit to use at the first sign of trouble. This would not be a substitute for proper veterinary attention, but would help control the signs in a crisis.

A SWOLLEN EYE

The eye itself may swell as a result of injury within the eye or something pushing the eyeball out of its normal place. Either way it is potentially serious, so if the eye looks significantly bigger than normal, consult your vet within 24 hours. It is much more common for the tissues around the eye to swell than the eye itself. A horse may have a swelling around the eye in the same way as a human develops a 'black eye'. Providing the eye itself is not painful, you can treat the swelling with ice packs and cold compresses. Contact your vet if the swelling does not reduce in size within a few days or becomes painful.

A CLOSED EYE

This is an indication of pain. It may mean there is something in the eye or there is an underlying painful condition such as moon blindness.

- Never try to force the eye open. Try to look inside by standing on the side of the bad eye and making a sound, e.g. whistling, so your horse will look at you. If his eye is not too sore, he will open it to look at you, especially if you do this out of bright light.
- If you see a foreign body trapped under the eyelids, such as a long hair or a grass seed, do not try and pull it out, but seek professional help from your vet. It is very easy to damage the delicate surface of the eye whilst removing a foreign body, especially if the horse moves. It is, however, usually safe to remove dirt and debris from the corner of the eye.

BLINDNESS

Horses can suddenly go blind in either one or both eyes. Most commonly this will happen as a result of a blow to the head, particularly if the horse rears up and falls over backwards. The eye itself may not appear to be damaged, but a knock to the head can cause damage to the nerves and parts of the brain that control the horse's ability to see.

It can be difficult to tell how well a horse can see. If he is blind in only one eye, a horse is often remarkably good at compensating with his good eye. Look for the following signs:

- A horse which is bumping into things, stepping very cautiously and twitching his ears a lot as he tries to listen to make up for not being able to see. It can still be hard to tell, particularly if the horse has just got up after a fall and is weak and wobbly anyway.
- If your horse is not weak and wobbly, but you are still uncertain if he can see, try leading the horse through stable doorways, gates and around obstacles such as hay bales and buckets to see if he can avoid them safely. See if he can cope with an obstacle course with both eyes. Then try blindfolding one eye and repeating the exercise to see if each eye is functional.
- Try throwing rolled up tissues or cotton wool balls at the horse and see if there is a response.

If you are in any doubt, make an appointment to see your vet. If your horse has recently suffered a blow to the head and appears weak, wobbly or visually impaired, you should contact your vet straightaway.

First aid measures for a blind horse include ensuring he is kept in safe, ideally familiar, surroundings, such as his own stable if he is at home, or another box with nothing he can injury himself on since he cannot see any hazards. Remember he will not be able to see his food or water, so will need help. He will also be frightened, so talk to him reassuringly so he knows that you are there.

Foaling emergencies

See page 101.

A very thickened
leg as a result of
infection. This is a
case of lymphangitis

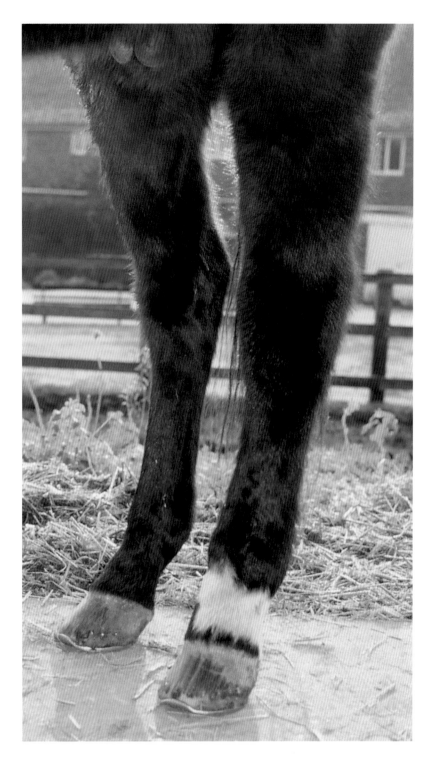

Filled legs

Filled legs are more likely to be serious if only one leg is involved. Horses commonly develop a localised infection involving just one leg. This is frequently because of a wound on that leg. Sometimes there is an obvious area of broken skin where infection has entered. For instance, a patch of mud fever on the heels can cause the whole leg to swell. A tiny puncture wound is another possible cause and it can be hard to identify without clipping the hair. Occasionally an unidentified abscess, e.g. pus in the foot, will cause swelling up the leg. **Cellulitis** is the technical term for infection within the tissues, which can result in swelling up the leg to above the knee or hock. In very severe cases, where the lymphatic system is involved, it is termed **lymphangitis**.

- If the horse is lame, in pain and has a raised temperature, an infection such as severe cellulitis or lymphangitis should be suspected. Your vet should be contacted the same day, since prompt treatment with appropriate antibiotics provides the best chance for a full recovery.

Other causes of a swollen leg include tendon injuries and localised tissue swelling known as **oedema**. Some cases need rest, e.g. tendon injuries, whereas others, e.g. oedema, need exercise to reduce the swelling. Your vet should be consulted within 48 hours if the leg does not reduce in size or before that if the horse is very lame. If in doubt, rest the horse until your vet has examined him thoroughly.

- If the horse is otherwise well, shows no sign of lameness and has been stabled for any length of time, it is likely that this swelling is as a result of poor circulation to the lower limbs. This means that his legs will fill if he is kept confined, particularly if he is on a rich diet. It will affect all four legs or both front and both back legs, not just one leg on its own. This sort of swelling will go down with exercise. If the swelling remains or increases after exercise then contact your vet.

Foreign bodies

Foreign bodies are a first aid dilemma. If a foreign body is wedged in a wound, in most circumstances it is best left there until you have veterinary help, unless it is very loose. In the majority of cases, particularly with wood in feet, a foreign body can be wedged in very hard and be extremely difficult and potentially painful to remove. It is much better to do this with a vet who can administer appropriate painkillers and sedatives to the horse and then check the injury properly. Another concern is that a foreign body may have broken off within a wound, so the site of the accident and any potential foreign bodies, e.g. broken fencing, should be noted. It is not uncommon for a piece of wood to break off deep within a wound and only be discovered months later, when the wound fails to heal.

This horse managed to get a foreign body (i.e. a piece of fence) in his forehead

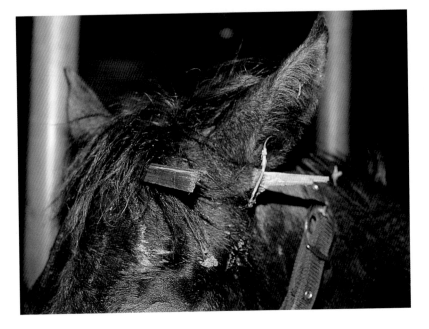

Foreign bodies in the foot

The one exception to this rule is when a nail is stuck in the sole of the foot. This should be removed if the horse is trying to weight-bear, to prevent the nail penetrating more deeply. The nail should be kept and your vet contacted immediately as a deep puncture wound in the foot can have life-threatening consequences. It is critical to note:

- where the nail penetrated the foot
- the angle at which it went in
- how deep it went in, i.e. the length of nail within the foot.

Ideally, if a nail is removed, mark the point it went in with an indelible marker pen. Shallow penetrations at the heel are least likely to cause any problems, but the deeper the nail goes the more dangerous it is, particularly if it happens to pierce the middle third of the foot. This is the real danger zone. If a nail or anything else has pierced the middle of the foot deeply, call your vet immediately. This is because several vital structures are located in the middle of the foot. These include:

- the navicular bone and associated structures
- the deep digital flexor tendon and its sheath
- the coffin joint.

Wounds that penetrate deep into the toe of a horse's foot may infect or break the pedal bone. Wounds in the heel tend to produce infection in the area of the puncture, but are rarely life-threatening.

The foot can be divided into three zones to assess the danger of a deep nail penetration. Shallow penetrations are unlikely to touch any vital structures. Deep penetration in **zone 1** may damage the pedal bone. **Zone 3**, at the back of the heel, would require a very long nail or other foreign body to strike the deep digital flexor tendon and cause serious damage. The middle of the foot, **zone 2**, is the **danger zone** as vital structures lie just over the frog. (a) Section through the foot; (b) ground surface of the foot

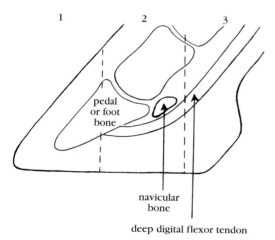

(a) Section through the foot

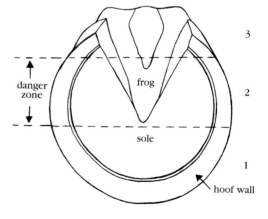

(b) Ground surface of the foot

71

If a dirty foreign body, such as a nail, reaches any of these vital structures, major treatment is needed to eliminate infection. Poulticing is unlikely to be sufficient. To maximise the chance of returning the horse to soundness you must contact your vet, who will need to undertake aggressive diagnostic measures and treatment right away. Punctures to the foot can be misleading (in that they can look so much better when the nail is removed) so that treatment may be delayed until it is too late. In these cases pain is not always a clear indicator that something is seriously wrong. With a nail puncture that goes more than 2 cm (1 in) into the foot, do not delay before contacting your vet.

What your vet will do

This will depend on the individual case. In the majority of deep nail punctures to the foot, X-ray pictures will be taken using either a sterile metal probe or some contrast agent (a liquid which shows up on an X-ray when it is injected down the hole left by the nail). It can be hard sometimes to locate the hole, particularly if the original nail wound is in the frog, as this will tend to close up once the nail has been pulled out.

Once it is established where exactly the nail went, an appropriate method of treatment can be selected. Deep wounds involving vital structures will need serious surgery to open up

Left: A puncture in the foot being explored with a metal probe to find out how deep it is

Right: A metal probe within a puncture wound in the foot on an X-ray picture. In this case the consequences are serious as the tip of the probe touched the navicular bone

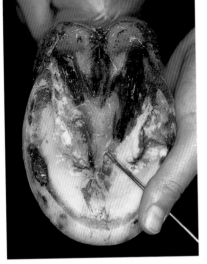

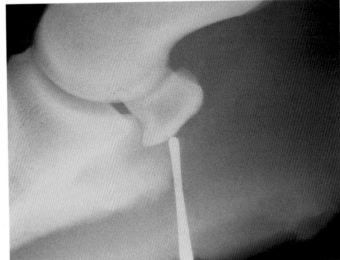

and clean the contaminated area. If the navicular bursa is involved, a window may be cut in the bottom of the foot under general anaesthesia to allow drainage. This is called a 'streetnail procedure'. Other cases are treated by arthroscopy, where a tiny telescope is inserted into the bursa, again under general anaesthesia, to assess and repair the damage. Large doses of powerful antibiotics are also needed. Even then, with all available treatment, the outlook can be poor. The chance of a successful recovery is maximised by starting treatment as soon as possible after the original injury.

Lameness, sudden and severe

If your horse suddenly goes very lame, look carefully at the foot first. If this happens out on a ride, get off immediately, take the reins over his head and have a look. Everyone dreads a broken bone, but do remember that most lameness is due to something in the foot rather than a fracture. Check the foot first to make sure the horse has not simply trodden on a stone. A badly fitting shoe can slip and cause pain. Many sprains and strains will ease within a short period of time, and you may then be able gently to move your horse to shelter and seek help.

Lameness may require urgent treatment. I am often amazed how some people will wait days before calling a vet for a horse that is hopping lame, whilst others will consider the slightest degree of lameness to be a dire emergency. In general, if a horse is standing on only three legs and cannot walk, you should contact your vet straightaway. Whereas, if a horse can walk on the lame leg, but prefers to rest it, it is less critical, but would still be best to be seen by a vet the same day. When a horse has suddenly become noticeably lame, for instance overnight or following a wound, it is sensible to contact your vet the same day. It is harder to know when a gradually worsening lameness becomes a serious problem. Certainly, if it does not respond to a few days' rest or cannot be resolved by your farrier checking the foot, then it is time to call the vet.

Suspected fractures

If a horse cannot put any weight on the injured leg at all, or is standing oddly, you will need to get help to wherever the horse is rather than make your horse hop home. A broken leg can occur in many different situations and should be suspected when:

- a horse is suddenly seen to be non-weight-bearing lame, i.e. he cannot use the leg at all
- a loud crack is heard prior to the onset of lameness
- the limb is totally unstable and may bend at an unusual angle
- the horse is in extreme pain.

In such circumstances the horse will be shocked and feel cold, so try to cover him with any coat or rug that is to hand. Keep him quiet till help arrives. If a horse is found like this in the field, do not attempt to move him, but put a headcollar on and hold him still, so that he does not try to move on the injured limb. It is movement which makes the horse distressed as he realises he cannot use the leg, so keep any suspected fracture as still as you can. Food is often a good way of calming a horse: hay and a bucket of feed are good emergency painkillers in many such cases.

- Contact your vet immediately, requesting immediate emergency attention, and explain why, so that the vet knows the potential seriousness of the situation.
- To save time when the vet arrives, try and organise transport in advance so everything is ready if the horse has to be moved. Horses with a leg injury may find it easier to walk up a gentle trailer ramp than a steeper one into a horsebox. Racecourses and other equine facilities have special horse ambulances for just this purpose. If a horse with a broken leg is to be travelled, the way in which this is done can make an enormous difference to the final outcome. A good supporting splint and an easy journey with a good driver can help reduce the chance of further destabilising the broken bones.

Regrettably, many fractures in the horse are untreatable, particu-

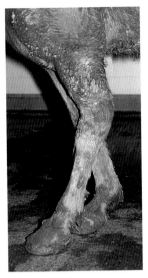

This pony has a fractured radius, i.e. a broken bone involving the upper forelimb. It can be seen that the pony is standing oddly, with no weight on the injured limb

larly those where there is an open wound with the bone visible through the skin. In these cases the tissue damage and infection will be overwhelming. The majority of broken long bones of the upper hind and forelimb will also be impossible to repair. Other lower limb fractures are potentially repairable, but you and your horse will be facing a long and costly course of surgical treatment. In many cases it is kindest if the horse can be euthanised (i.e. put to sleep) as soon as possible. If you are not the owner, try to contact them so that they are available to discuss the situation with the vet.

Having said that, every year vets are called to many suspected fractures which turn out to be relatively easily repairable bone chips rather than complete fractures, or other causes of sudden severe lameness, such as pus in the foot or a locking patella. So do not despair. Obtain immediate veterinary help and an accurate diagnosis as soon as possible.

Pus in the foot

Foot pain is one of the commonest causes of lameness in the horse. The most frequent, which sometimes appears suddenly, is pus in the foot. This is properly called a **sub-solar abscess**. This is particularly common in wet weather, when moisture, dirt and bacteria track up through tiny cracks in the hoof. Infection then rapidly develops, with a build up of pus within the confines of the hoof, which is extremely painful for the horse.

What to look for

In the early stages there may be only a slight lameness which can progress to a state where it is so sore that the horse will not put the foot to the ground, i.e. he is literally hopping lame. Also there may be:

- increased heat in the foot, i.e. that hoof may feel hotter than the others
- increased pulse to the foot, as with laminitis but affecting only the one foot
- pain and discomfort

- swelling up the leg, so this may be mistaken for a tendon injury
- pus discharging from the coronary band. If the abscess is not drained it will burst out from the coronary band.

What to do about it

If you suspect your horse has pus in the foot, you should contact your vet or your farrier to attend to the horse as soon as possible. The cure is to drain the abscess, which will usually involve removing the shoe. Once the abscess has been located and the pus drained out, the horse will immediately feel very much better.

First aid treatment includes putting on a poultice to encourage the abscess to drain. A poultice on the sole of the foot (see bandaging the foot, page 37) when you first suspect the problem will help the horse feel more comfortable. This will soften the hard horn, making the vet's or farrier's job of paring down with a hoof knife easier. You should avoid poulticing around the coronary band because, firstly, a hot poultice will burn the skin, and, secondly, it is best to encourage the infection to drain downwards rather than burst open at the coronary band.

Once the abscess has drained, the whole foot should be

Left: When the pressure from an abscess within the foot builds up, it can burst open and discharge as pus from the coronary band (arrowed)

Right: If a horse has pus in his foot, the infection may also drain from the sole, particularly when the abscess is opened as here (arrowed)

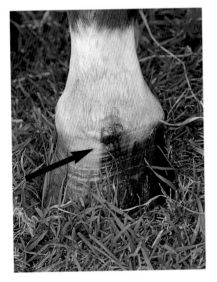

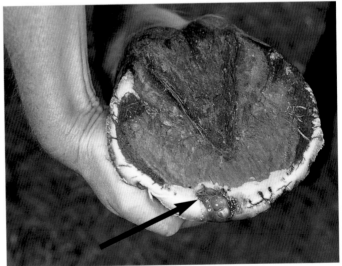

cleaned. Sometimes soaking the foot in a tub of warm water with a little table salt or Epsom salts will help the horse and clean the foot. The vet or farrier will advise you on how to clean the actual area of the abscess. It may need to be flushed with hydrogen peroxide or an antiseptic to reduce the infection. It is then important that it is kept poulticed or protected with some sort of antiseptic dressing until it has healed sufficiently to prevent further dirt entering the area of damage.

It is also important to ensure the horse is up to date with his tetanus vaccinations.

A horse with pus in the foot is best kept stabled, particularly when the foot is bandaged.

Eight out of ten lamenesses originate in the foot, the ninth is also likely to be in the foot but you just cannot find it and only the tenth will be somewhere else on the leg altogether.

Other foot lameness

As well as pus in the foot, there are other causes of sudden severe lameness involving the foot. These include a **bruise**, which will show similar symptoms to pus in the foot. A **corn** is a bruise that appears specifically at the area known as the **seat of corn** on the foot, i.e. between the frog and the hoof wall. These problems are hard to differentiate from an abscess. If in doubt you should ask your vet to see the horse within the next 24 hours or so. The best first aid is to keep the horse confined to a box so he can rest the sore foot. Cleaning the foot and poulticing it may be of benefit whilst you obtain professional help.

The best prevention for all these feet problems is regular trimming and shoeing to keep the foot in good condition.

Accidents associated with shoeing

On rare occasions, a horse will go severely lame soon after shoeing. Although not anywhere near as bad as a fracture, this can be a cause for alarm. It should be remembered that shoeing horses is a very skilled job. Sometimes a horseshoe nail will touch the sensitive tissues of the foot and the horse will be temporarily lame. It is known as **nail bind** or a **pricked foot**. This is more likely to happen if the horse is badly behaved and will not stand still for the farrier or it has particularly poor feet with thin hooves.

A section through a foot to show the normal positioning of a horse shoe nail (a) and when the nail is too close to the sensitive laminae, causing pain and lameness (b)

WHAT TO DO

Ask your farrier to check the foot and remove the shoe if needed.

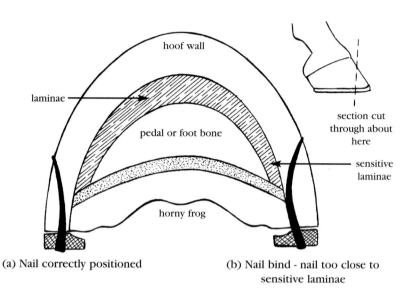

hoof wall

laminae

pedal or foot bone

horny frog

section cut through about here

sensitive laminae

(a) Nail correctly positioned

(b) Nail bind - nail too close to sensitive laminae

Upward fixation of the patella

This is included here as it is a cause of sudden severe lameness which is sometimes mistaken for a broken leg. This is when one of the back legs becomes stuck out behind the horse, or as more commonly seen, in a pony. The animal may hop forward, dragging the toe along the ground. It is commonly called a 'locking patella' because the patella or kneecap catches over the main bones of the upper hind limb. This is a normal part of the equine mechanism for sleeping standing up. Normally the horse can unlock or free the patella, but in these cases it catches. Consequently, the leg may appear stuck at an odd angle, hence the confusion with a fracture.

WHAT TO DO ABOUT IT

Look carefully and establish that the leg is stuck backward rather than hanging at an odd angle as with a fracture. Also, in these cases the animal is rarely distressed. Frequently, the patella will unlock of its own accord after a few strides. If not, it is often possible make it shift by:

- making the horse jump forward
- making the horse go back
- manipulating the stifle.

The condition is most commonly seen in immature, unfit or poorly muscled animals who will do this same thing repeatedly, e.g. every morning, as they come out of their stable. The condition will frequently improve as the horse grows older and stronger. However, if the problem persists you should make an appointment to see your vet as some cases will require surgery.

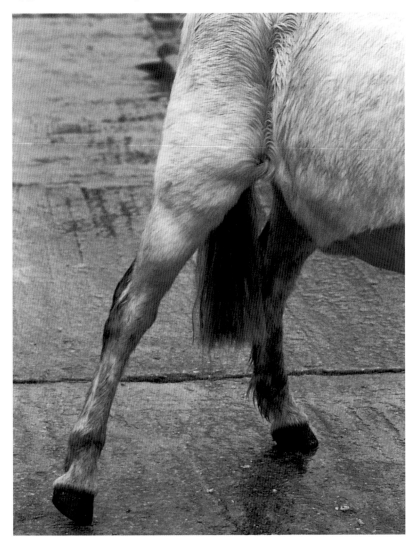

Upward fixation of the patella: a hind leg sticks out backwards and the toe is dragged

Other sudden severe lameness

Many other problems can cause sudden severe lameness (e.g. see tendon injuries page 98 and wounds page 24). In all cases the basic principles of first aid should be followed:

- The horse should be restrained, so that it cannot damage itself further.
- If the horse is in pain and cannot stand on the limb, immediate veterinary help should be sought.

Laminitis

Laminitis is a very painful condition, most commonly seen in overweight ponies grazing lush grass. It can also affect larger horses, particularly if they are already ill for another reason, e.g. a mare that has had a retained placenta and other problems after foaling. **Acute laminitis** is the early stage of the condition when the horse or pony is uncomfortable and showing lameness but major changes have not yet happened within the foot. This is an *emergency* and proper treatment needs to be started at once to prevent serious damage.

Chronic laminitis occurs when the pedal bone has rotated or sunk or if the condition has been going on for more than 48 hours. These cases are not necessarily such an immediate emergency, but once you have noticed a problem you should contact your vet soon, preferably the same day if the horse or pony is in pain. If acute laminitis is caught in the early stages, it can prevent long-term problems. So, particularly when you are faced with what appears to be a new case of laminitis, you should treat it as an emergency and contact your vet as soon as possible.

What to look for?

In severe cases of laminitis, the feet are so painful that the horse or pony cannot stand or is unable to move. The laminitis case may tremble and look stressed and anxious.

The feet are usually hot and the horse tends to stand with his

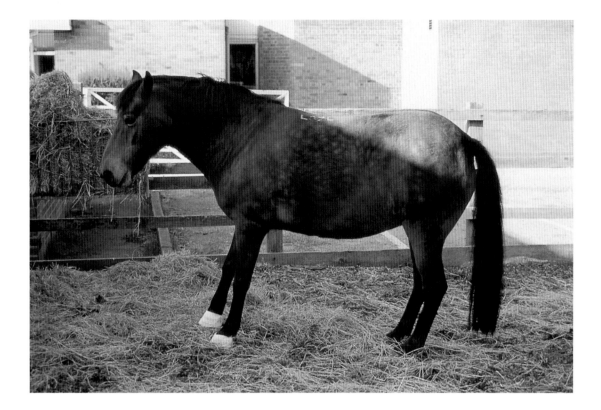

A pony with severe laminitis

legs stretched forward. Milder cases will be uncertain which foot to stand on, so they constantly shift their weight because whichever foot they stand on hurts. The intense pain associated with severe laminitis means the pulse and respiratory rate rise. Frequently an increased pulse is obvious where the digital artery runs over the fetlock. In severe laminitis cases, this digital pulse (which is where the blood going to the foot flows) will be pounding on all four feet.

Acute laminitis is usually easily recognised as the horse or pony is crippled, but the milder forms of chronic laminitis are less obvious and can be confused with other sorts of lameness. Signs include:

- intermittent lameness, especially on rough ground. Typically, this is the pony which is said to 'feel his feet'
- being footsore or lame after having the feet trimmed or reshod
- abnormal hoof growth seen as diverging rings around the hoof

81

wall, which are wider at the heel than at the toe. This will be associated with an abnormally shaped foot; characteristically long toes with overgrown heels

- the sole of the foot may drop because of the shift of the pedal bone, making the sole flatter. In the worst cases it will bulge out and actually be convex. The pedal bone may even drop through the sole
- pus in the foot (i.e. a foot abscess) is common because of the abnormally weak horn growth and the increased chance of infection developing in the diseased tissue of the foot
- a wider than normal white line at the ground surface. Frequently you can see red or pink areas of blood staining (from the diseased laminae) particularly when the farrier trims the feet. This is a weakness and again increases the chances of infection
- ponies that have had previously had laminitis often have thick cresty necks where fat deposits have accumulated and these may persist even when they lose weight elsewhere.

What to do about it?

Rapid treatment increases the chance of a successful outcome, so never 'wait and see' with laminitis. The very painful cases need to see a vet as soon as possible; the mild chronic cases can be carefully managed by your vet and farrier working together.

FIRST AID ACTION FOR LAMINITIS

If you think your horse or pony has laminitis, never force him to walk but allow him to lie down if he wishes to do so. The most helpful thing to do is minimise the pain, as the more pain there is the more stressed the horse or pony will be and the worse the laminitis will become. So try to keep him calm and quiet. You will need strong painkillers from your vet to help, but keeping the patient still until the vet arrives will be useful. If the feet are very hot, standing them in cold water or hosing will provide temporary relief. This should only be done as a short-term measure, however, as it may further compromise the blood supply to the foot. It is now thought that warm water hosing or applying warm water compresses around the lower limbs (e.g. warm wet towels) is actually more beneficial, followed by bandaging the limbs to prevent swelling and help to keep blood in the foot area. It is possible to tape frog supports onto the feet to help. Various types are available, ranging from rubber wedges, bandage rolls or purpose-made styrofoam pads. It is best that these are fitted in conjunction with advice from your vet or farrier to ensure that they are put on properly.

Unfortunately, prevention is far better than first aid for laminitis cases. When the problem develops as a complication of another condition, prevention is obviously difficult. In the overweight or overfed animal, a carefully controlled diet, increased exercise and good regular farriery are the obvious, but not easy, answers.

Nosebleeds (epistaxis)

Nosebleeds (properly known as epistaxis) do occur in horses and are frequently due to trauma to the head.

- A slight bleed from one nostril, which stops in fifteen minutes, is unlikely to be serious but your vet should be contacted if it recurs. Recurrent nosebleeds should always be investigated.

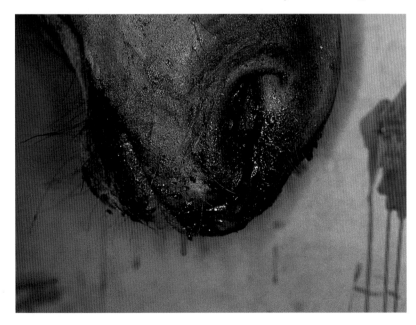

This horse was found in his stable having had a severe nosebleed (note the blood on the stable wall). This case was due to a fall in the box in which the horse had hit his head and broken a bone within the nose

- A moderate nosebleed accompanied by coughing suggests a foreign body wedged in the nose or throat. This, or a copious nosebleed, is a true emergency and your vet should be contacted immediately, particularly if the horse is distressed.

Whilst waiting for the vet the horse should be kept as calm as possible. The nose should not be packed as horses breathe only through their noses, so this would distress him. It may help to hold an ice pack just below the horse's eyes. If the bleeding is coming from inside the nose area, this can help slow it down. A nose bleed is one of the times to remember that horses have very large volumes of blood inside them, so what looks like a lot coming out of the nose may not be critical for the horse. Even so, it cannot be allowed to continue for more than fifteen minutes. If it does your vet should be consulted as an emergency. It may help your vet if you can tell him or her if the bleeding is just from one nostril, which means it is coming from inside the nose area, or from both nostrils, which means it is more likely to originate somewhere further back.

What the vet will do

Again this depends on the individual case. The cause of a small, one-off nosebleed may never be found, but recurrent or persistent nosebleeds may well require endoscopy (i.e. an examination of the inside of the nose and throat with a flexible instrument that enables the vet to see what is going on inside). X-ray pictures may also help to examine the skull. There are some serious, but rare, conditions in the horse, which start as tiny nosebleeds that then get worse and worse, so always have a significant nosebleed checked out promptly.

Poisoning

Poisoning is frequently suspected by owners as a cause of any unexplained illness in their horse or pony. In fact, poisoning is an unusual cause of sudden illness, although it may explain more long-term illness, including weight loss, inappetance and nervous signs which are associated with ragwort poisoning, amongst others. It is important to remember that there is no toxin screen that can test for all possible poisons. If poisoning is suspected, all possible clues should be considered to establish what is the most likely cause.

Realistically, poisoning may be suspected if:
- many horses are sick at once with no known infectious cause
- the affected individual(s) have been exposed to a new environment, e.g. new grazing
- there has been a recent change in feed
- the affected horse(s) has insufficient grazing or feed so is more likely to nibble something else
- very unusual clinical signs are seen that cannot be otherwise explained
- an unexplained death has occurred.

If you do suspect a possible poisoning, particularly if a horse has died suddenly, your vet should be called straightaway. Immediate action should include preventing further exposure to the poison, e.g. take horses off the field where there is a suspected problem or stop feeding a suspected feed. Your vet will be able to advise you on further action. He or she will have access to the National Poisons Unit, who can give specialist advice on the correct antidote for a particular poison if one is available. Initially, treatment of any horse suspected of poison may include efforts to reduce absorption of poison, e.g. by administering activated charcoal, or to hasten the elimination of a poison, e.g. by administration of liquid paraffin. You should keep the horse warm and comfortable during treatment.

There are a large number of potentially poisonous plants in the UK. The majority are not actually palatable to horses, so they will only eat them if nothing else is available or if the plants are cut and wilted, when they may taste more acceptable. Ragwort is a good example. It is rarely eaten if growing on the pasture, but will be eaten in hay.

It is sensible to check your pasture before you have a problem.

The most common poisonous plants found in the UK

Common name	Proper name	Common name	Proper name
Acacia (false)	*Robinia pseudoacacia*	Oak	*Quercus* spp.
Box	*Buxus sempervivens*	Onions (domestic)	*Allium cepa*
Bracken	*Pteridum aquilinum*	Peas (sweet/wild)	*Lathyrus* spp.
Buckwheat	*Fagoptrum esculentum*	Potato (green or rotten)	*Solanum tuberosum*
Buttercups	*Ranunculus* spp.	Privet	*Ligustrum* spp.
Cherry	*Prunus* spp.	Ragwort	*Senecio* spp.
Foxglove	*Digitalis* spp.	Red maple	*Acer rubrum*
Groundsel	*Senecio vulgaris*	Rhododendron	*Rhododendron ponticum*
Hemlock	*Conium maculatum*	Rhubarb	*Rheum cultorum*
Henbane	*Hyoscyamus niger*	Scottish broom	*Cystisus scoparius*
Horse chestnut	*Aesculus hippocastum*	St John's wort	*Hypericum perforatum*
Horsetail	*Equisetum* spp.	Thorn-apple	*Datura stramonium*
Hydrangea	*Hydrangea* spp.	Tobacco plant	*Nicotiana* spp.
Laburnum	*Laburnum anagyroides*	Water dropwort	*Oenanthe* spp.
Laurel	*Prunus* spp.	Water hemlock	*Cicuta virosa*
Lily of the valley	*Convallaria majalis*	Wild onions	*Allium* spp.
Marijuana (hemp)	*Cannabis sativa*	Yew	*Taxus* spp.
Nightshade	*Atropa belladona*		

This list of poisonous plants does not include all possiblities, and some of those that are listed are significantly less poisonous than others. Buttercups and bracken, for instance, can be extremely poisonous but are rarely eaten in sufficiently large quantities to cause a problem as they taste unpleasant, so the horse will tend to ignore them. Horses are quite picky eaters and will tend to nibble around and avoid things that they do not like. Conversely, all parts of the yew are highly poisonous but also very palatable. Horses are extremely susceptible to the toxin. About 150 g of leaves are sufficient to kill a horse, which is basically one horse-sized mouthful. As it is a well-recognised poisonous plant, it is rarely found bordering pastures, however horses may grab some to eat when out at exercise. If your horse does this, you should immediately pull the leaves out of his mouth. There is no antidote, so avoidance is the only safe approach.

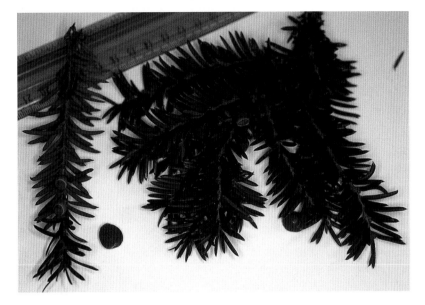

Yew is very poisonous

Pus in the foot

See lameness sudden and severe, page 73.

Retained placenta

See page 118.

Skin rashes

Skin rashes are rarely an emergency. Occasionally **urticaria (nettle rash** or **hives)** can produce a dramatic allergic reaction with raised patches all over the skin. You will see lumps of all different sizes appearing rapidly under your horse's skin, rather like those you would see on yourself if you fell in a nettle patch. The skin

Urticaria or nettle rash can suddenly appear as lumps anywhere on the horse's head, body or limbs

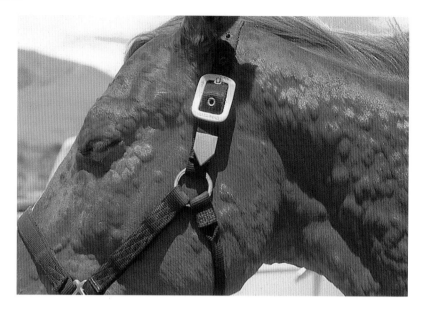

lesions develop rapidly and will often disappear within a few hours. They start as small bumps which spread together into larger, doughy areas of swelling.

What causes this?

Urticaria is the result of an allergic reaction to something. It can be hard to determine what. In many cases you will never establish what was the cause. It will be something to which the horse has previously been exposed and become sensitive to, so that his body reacts to it. Possibilities include pollens, insect bites, insect repellents or other topical treatments such as shampoos, or drugs which have been given to your horse.

You should call the vet if:

- the horse is distressed or the breathing is laboured
- the eyelids and muzzle are very swollen
- there is no improvement after 24 hours.

A large number of cases will clear up without treatment and never happen again. If the condition does happen more than once, you should consult your vet in case there is a risk of a more serious allergy.

Occasionally a horse will fall or roll into nettles. In a thin-skinned Thoroughbred type this is very uncomfortable and the horse will be very distressed by it. If it were not for the nettle rash and often the circumstantial evidence of squashed nettles nearby, it would be easy to think it was something much more serious. The horse may look very lame, weak and wobbly or repeatedly turn round to look at his flank as if he had colic. The condition should settle down rapidly, but if it persists contact your vet.

Ringworm is another skin rash which may be considered an emergency by the horse's owner although it is not painful and will not upset the horse. The reason why people take it seriously is that it is very infectious. It can spread rapidly from horse to horse, or from horse to human, but it is *never* fatal and in truth cannot be considered to be a genuine emergency.

Ringworm is a fungal infection of the skin. Confusingly, despite the name, ringworm is not always ring-shaped and has nothing to do with worms! There are many different types of ringworm, but the two main ones are *Trichophyton* and *Microsporum* species. The fungus grows across the surface of the skin and around the hairs, producing a variety of changes affecting the horse's coat and skin.

What to look for

Often all that is noticed in the early stages is tufts of hair that may appear raised up from the rest of the coat with a slight swelling underneath. People imagine ringworm patches to be circular, but in fact they can be any shape. Usually the tufts of affected hair fall out, leaving the skin underneath looking somewhat raw and sore. Classically, ringworm develops into grey, flaking areas with broken hairs. The coat will then gradually regrow over the next month. Remember that ringworm can appear in many different disguises. Any skin rash or sore or bald area for which there is no other obvious explanation should be checked for ringworm. When in doubt, ringworm is one of the few conditions for which it may be best to treat anyway to avoid any risk of infection spreading further.

Ringworm can appear anywhere on the body, but the most common site for it is where the skin is in contact with tack or

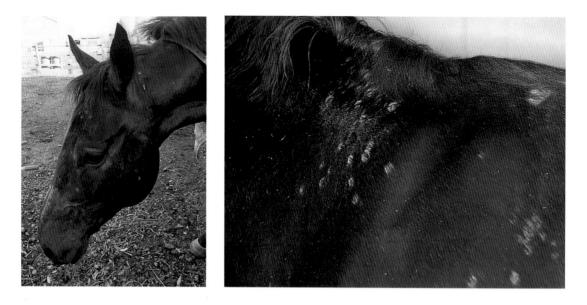

Left: Ringworm rash can appear in many different forms

Right: Ringworm rash can be scattered all over the horse's body, as here

harness, such as the saddle or girth areas. Here the skin is rubbed and tiny abrasions develop through which the fungus invades. Young horses are said to be more at risk, probably because they have less immunity. Older horses usually show milder signs of ringworm and recover more quickly.

Horses do not die from ringworm so there is no need to consider it as a crisis, but it is important to be aware that ringworm is highly contagious. It can spread very rapidly from one horse to another unless sensible precautions are taken to stop it. It spreads either by direct contact or on grooming kit or tack, buckets or rugs. Worst of all, the ringworm fungus will produce spores that can remain dormant on woodwork for over a year. This means that stables and fencing can become contaminated which is why some horses are unfortunate enough to develop ringworm when put in a stable which has been empty for ages. Equally, it is a very good reason not to share tack, particularly girths which, by rubbing and getting damp and sweaty, are the ideal way for ringworm to spread!

What to do if you suspect ringworm

If you suspect ringworm on a horse, sensible control measures include:

- keeping any suspected case separate in his own box; if an infected horse is isolated in his stable he should not spread the disease provided he cannot touch other horses. Crowded stable yards are always a greater risk
- do not groom or clip an affected horse because of the risk of spreading spores
- avoid riding an affected horse. This reduces the chance of spread and prevents the skin sores becoming worse as the tack rubs them
- do not share rugs, tack or grooming kit
- ask your vet to check any suspected case to obtain a diagnosis
- do not delay treatment of *both* the horse and his surroundings.

Your vet may be able to diagnose ringworm from looking at the skin lesions, particularly if several horses are involved. Lab tests may be needed for confirmation.

Horses can catch the infection from other animals, particularly cattle, dogs or wild animals, but can also pass it on to people. It is one of the few conditions you can catch from your horse, so for that reason alone it needs to be considered seriously. If you have a horse with even a mild skin irritation and you also develop a skin rash, seek medical advice. Autumn, winter and early spring are the most common seasons for outbreaks.

Control of ringworm

The incubation period for ringworm is between one and four weeks. Most cases, if left, will eventually clear up on their own, but it is best treated to avoid further spread.

The aim of treatment is twofold: firstly to kill the fungus and secondly to destroy the infective spores. It is important to cure the infected horse, but also vital to reduce the environmental contamination. To treat the horse, there are some effective washes which can be sprayed or sponged onto the skin. The thick, crusting lesions and the hair coat usually make the application of a cream impractical. Your vet will be able to dispense the best treatment for your particular case. Antifungal powders may be prescribed to be fed to the horse. Care must be taken in using this in-feed medication, as it is dangerous for pregnant women or mares. If there is any risk it is best avoided, as the condition can usually be cured without resort to such drugs in the feed.

Isolating affected horses and ponies as much as possible is very important to limit environmental contamination. Any stables involved should be thoroughly cleaned and dirty bedding burnt. You should disinfect the rugs, fences and anything else a ringworm case has contacted. The need to do this is the biggest inconvenience with ringworm. However, one intensive attack on everything can reduce the spread amongst horses in the area. Remember that the wooden walls of most stables can harbour the ringworm spores all too easily. A variety of effective compounds can be used on tack, rugs and grooming kit without causing damage. Environmental treatment may include five to ten per cent bleach for concrete and creosote for wood. If there is a large area to be treated, it is possible to use horticultural foggers containing anti-fungal agents. This is very useful for items such as your best rug and saddle that cannot be treated with harsh disinfectant. Ask your vet for advice.

Shock

Shock is the response of a horse or human to trauma, pain and infection. It is a serious condition in itself, which can pull a patient into a downward spiral, reducing their chances of recovery. Remember that horses do not have the human capacity for reasoning and so will be frightened by things which we understand and therefore do not fear. Reassuring and calming a horse can help whilst appropriate veterinary attention is sought.

Signs to look for:

- shaking and shivering
- rapid breathing
- a weak pulse
- pale mucous membranes
- cold extremities: in the horse, feeling the ears is always a good guide.

The signs of shock result from disturbances of the circulation as a result of an accident, injury or illness. Causes can include loss of blood and dehydration as well as overwhelming infection. The body's natural responses can be counterproductive and the damage becomes self-perpetuating and potentially disastrous.

What you should do whilst you wait for the vet

Keep the horse calm and quiet. If it is cold, bring him into a warm box and rug him up. If it is hot make sure he is not overheated. Try to keep him cool. Make sure there is water available for him to drink. Always warm a horse with extra rugs rather than closing up his stable, which will simply make the environment stuffy and airless.

What your vet will do

Treatment for shock very much depends on what is the cause. The vet will concentrate on establishing and controlling the primary cause of the shock. Many horses with severe colic will become shocked. In such cases it is important to treat the underlying colic as well as the signs of shock. Serious infections can cause shock, so antibiotic and other drugs may also be used. If the horse is bleeding, the cause has to be found and then stopped. Supportive treatment for severe shock will include administration of fluids. If the horse cannot drink, this can

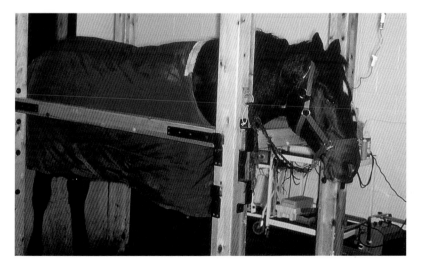

A sick horse suffering from shock being treated with intravenous fluids

93

require the administration of 40 to 80 litres of sterile fluids per day via an intravenous drip to combat the signs of shock. This will require intensive treatment in a hospital situation.

Strangles

Strangles is a highly infectious disease of horses which causes panic amongst horse and yard owners. It is not a genuine first aid problem but can be a major nuisance in curtailing equine activity.

Basically, strangles is a 'head cold' or throat infection caused by the bacterium *Streptococcus equi*. Mild cases may show no more than a runny nose and will recover within days, but severe strangles can lead to high temperature, depression, swollen glands and pus-filled abscesses. Historically the name strangles relates to the fact that bad cases produce abscesses around the throat area, which can affect the breathing and appear almost to strangle the horse. The disease can be fatal, but these days very few cases are that bad. Many cases show only as a mild respiratory infection.

An unjustified stigma accompanies strangles. When a yard is hit by strangles, the owners are sometimes blamed for the infection. This is both untrue and unfair. Strangles can strike those with the highest standards of care and management. Inevitably, as horses move and mix together, infections will spread, just like colds in people. One of the problems particular to strangles, however, is the occurrence of healthy long-term carriers, i.e. horses that carry the infection but show no signs of illness. This increases the spread of the disease.

What to look out for

It is impossible to tell if a horse is a carrier. Your vet may be able to do so with the aid of special laboratory tests. Signs of the disease may include:

- a high temperature
- depression and loss of appetite
- a discharge from the nostrils
- swollen glands

- abscesses, usually in the throat region
- occasionally, a cough.

What to do about it

If you are concerned that you may have this infection among your horses, contact your vet as soon as possible. Early diagnosis and prompt action will reduce the spread of the disease. In the meantime, keep any horses with suspicious signs of the disease away from other horses. It is also a sensible precaution to keep the normal contacts of these horses in isolation until you know if you have a confirmed case of strangles. Do not allow new animals to enter the premises unless they, too, can be kept in isolation. Take special care to ensure that infection is not spread through handlers, shared water troughs, direct contact, bedding and such like. It has been shown that bacteria can persist on wood and other surfaces for up to 63 days.

The most important thing is to be aware that you cannot tell if a horse definitely has strangles by clinical examination. Laboratory tests are required for clear confirmation and more accurate tests are being developed all the time. It is important to

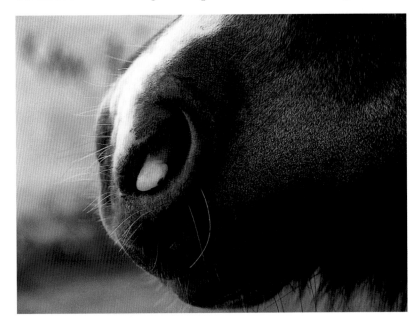

A thick yellow discharge of pus draining from the nose is a typical sign of strangles

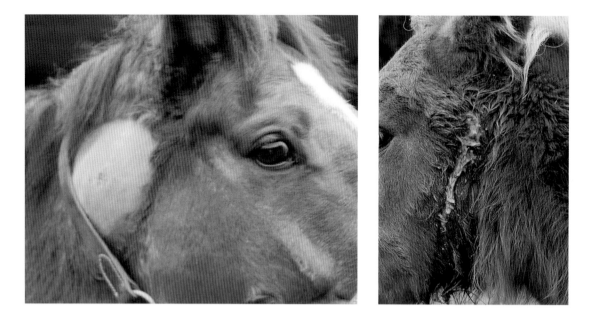

Left: A hot painful abscess in the glands around the head is another typical sign of strangles

Right: A burst abscess draining pus at this site is another typical sign of strangles

have an accurate diagnosis to be certain what you are dealing with and whether strict isolation is going to be properly justified.

Swellings

Swellings can appear anywhere on the body and can stem from a vast variety of causes. They should be taken seriously if they are painful, hot or rapidly enlarging, or associated with other signs of illness. Frequently such swellings are caused by abscesses. If a horse has recently had an injection, there may be a reaction or infection associated with that. Sometimes swellings are associated with the bacterial infection known as **strangles** and appear in the neck area.

• Your vet should be called the same day if you seriously suspect strangles and/or the horse is ill and has a swelling.

Large swellings can also appear due to trauma. These are due to giant blood blisters properly called haematoma. These can be bigger than a beach ball but are less serious than they look. They are neither hot nor painful.

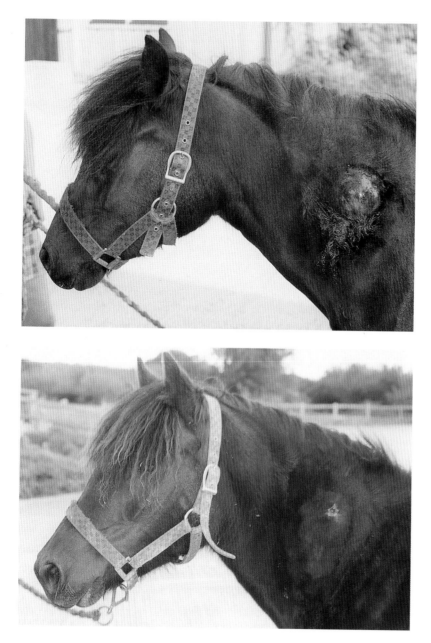

Top: A pony with a swelling on the neck. This is an abscess which is hot and painful to the touch and very inflamed, as compared to a haematoma

Bottom: The same pony with the abscess on the neck healing

- Your vet should be contacted if a significant swelling does not reduce in size after 48 hours.

Many different swellings can appear on the limbs. They are too numerous to describe here. In general, providing the horse is

97

A large haematoma on the stifle of the horse (arrowed). This is a sort of giant blood blister, which, in this case, formed after the horse had had a fall

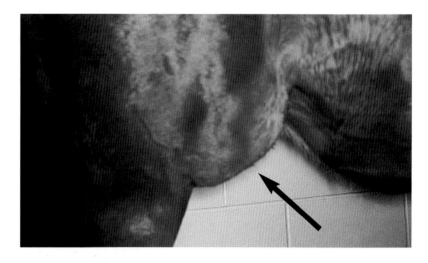

not severely lame, they do not merit urgent attention. If the swelling does not reduce in size, however, a routine appointment should be made to see your veterinary surgeon.

Tendon injuries

Tendon injuries require immediate first aid just like more obvious wounds. With a severe tendon injury, the horse may pull up lame or may develop heat and swelling, with or without lameness, soon after fast work. With less severe injuries there may be heat and swelling but no detectable lameness.

- As soon as possible, apply intense cold and support bandaging to reduce the inflammation. The aim of this is to minimise the damage to the tendon fibres and maximise the chance of a satisfactory repair. Proprietary chemical 'cooling' wraps are available to do this. In an emergency, packs of frozen peas, bags of ice or polystyrene cups filled with water and pre-frozen may be held against the limb. Cold treatment should be applied for a maximum of 30 minutes, followed by a 30-minute interval. This cycle can be repeated up to three times; any longer and you may cause yet more damage.
- If the fetlock has dropped close to the ground or the toe is pointing upwards, this indicates there is a major tendon rup-

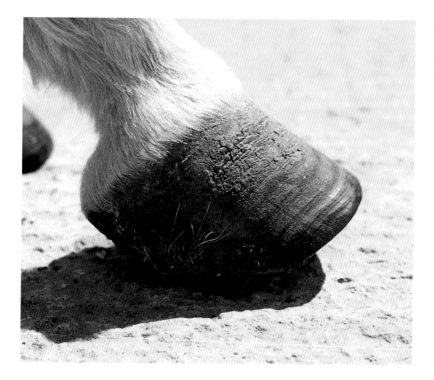

If the toe of the hoof does not touch the ground, as shown here, it means there is major tendon damage

ture and the vet should be contacted immediately.

- If there is an open wound or the horse is in severe pain, the vet should be contacted immediately.
- Immobilising the limb will prevent further damage and help relieve pain. You may need veterinary advice as to what is the best bandage to apply (see page 33).
- With any severe tendon injury it will help to make the horse feel better and reduce the amount of inflammatory damage if anti-inflammatory painkilling drugs can be given as soon as possible. Ideally, they should be administered directly into the vein by your vet, so that they start working straightaway. Powders taken by mouth in the feed will take longer to be effective.

If there is any suspicion of a tendon injury, the horse should be examined promptly by a vet before the horse returns to work. Even if the horse is not lame, significant tendon damage may have occurred. Diagnostic ultrasound scanning provides a very useful way of estimating the severity of a tendon injury.

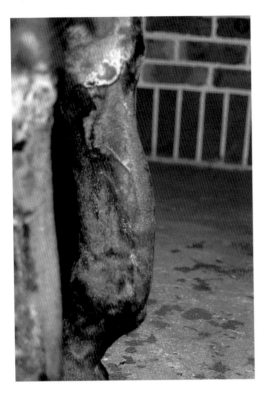

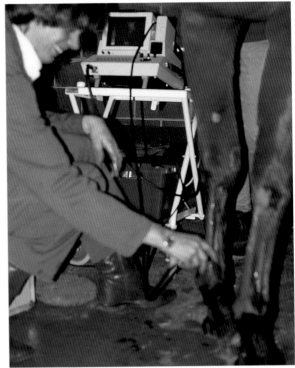

Left: A bowed tendon: this horse has sustained severe damage to the superficial flexor tendon

Right: Ultrasound scanning is a useful way for the vet to assess the severity of any tendon damage

Thumps

Thumps is the usual name for **synchronous diaphragmatic flutter**, which is a condition most likely to be seen in a dehydrated, exhausted horse towards the end of a competitive event, especially in hot, humid weather. It also occurs in heavy draught mares with foals at foot. The signs are a little like severe hiccups; the horse will breathe rapidly, with thumping sounds from the chest. At the same time the horse may sweat and appear uncomfortable, with muscle twitching and a stilted wobbly walk. In itself, 'thumps' is not harmful, but it is extremely disconcerting and is an indicator that there is a metabolic mix-up which should be sorted out.

- Thumps is caused by an electrolyte disturbance and the vet should be called immediately. With the correct treatment, such cases will rapidly improve.

6. WHAT TO DO WHEN FACED WITH BREEDING EMERGENCIES

Foaling emergencies

A foaling can be a number one, red alert emergency, but do remember that foaling is a *natural* process which usually results in the arrival of a live healthy foal without the need for human assistance or damage to the mare. The incidence of difficult births (i.e. **dystocia**) in the mare is said to be low (less than 4 per cent). On the rare occasion that things do go wrong, prompt and effective intervention is necessary and can make a critical difference between a live or dead mare and foal. It is best that your mare should foal down where there is experienced help to hand or that you should contact your vet as soon as foaling starts.

If you are uncertain of your abilities as a midwife, there is a strong case for sending your mare away to a stud where she can foal down under close professional supervision. If you do this, the mare should be taken to the premises where she is to foal about six weeks before full term. This allows the mare to become accustomed to any changes in management there. Importantly, it also ensures that her **colostrum** (i.e. first milk) will contain antibodies specific to those premises to help protect the foal.

Foaling facilities

If your mare is to foal down indoors, it is important to have a foaling box which is big enough for the mare to move around freely. The exact size will obviously depend on the size of the mare, but as a rough guide the average 500 kg Thoroughbred mare should have at least a 3.5 square metre foaling box. It is better to have it even bigger, if possible. This foaling box needs to be positioned so that the mare can be checked easily at night without disturbing her. Appropriate lighting is important. Ideally lights should be left on at a low level all night rather than switching them on and off every time the mare is checked. The bedding should be of the best straw (not shavings etc.), which is well banked up around the edges of the box.

At every foaling, those responsible should have available a basic first aid kit which should include:

- suitable antiseptic, e.g. povidine-iodine (i.e. Pevidine®) or chlorhexidine (i.e. Hibiscrub®) and warm water
- tail bandage for the mare
- sterile tape to tie the umbilical cord temporarily if needed
- sterile scissors to cut the cord if needed
- clean bucket and towels
- access to colostrum for the foal and replacement mare's milk, if needed: ask your vet what is best for you.

When will the mare foal?

Signs of impending foaling include:

- an enlarging abdomen
- development of the udder
- the presence of a watery or milky discharge from the teats. In most mares, a bead of colostrum (i.e. the first milk) dries at the teat end one to four days before foaling. This is called 'waxing up' because it looks somewhat like drips of wax from a candle
- relaxation of the sacrosciatic (pelvic) ligaments, which may

show as a softening of the hindquarters on either side of the tail
- lengthening of the vulva.

Unfortunately, mares vary tremendously in the signs they actually show. Many mares will not show any differences from normal whatsoever. For this reason the first some owners know about their foal's imminent birth is when they suddenly find a new arrival with the mare!

The normal length of gestation in the mare is 342 +/- 20 days. This means that you cannot rely on a mare to foal down at one predicted time and you could be checking her for many weeks before anything happens. There is a need to predict the time of foaling accurately. Anybody who has spent exhausting nights sitting up with mares waiting for them to foal will be well aware of this!

Warning devices

Many people use close circuit television systems to watch mares near to foaling, which is very helpful if you have the facilities and finance to do this. A cheap and basic alternative is to use a baby monitor, so you can at least listen in on your mare. A variety of foaling alarms are also available. In the UK, the most commonly used system is one which straps around the mare and sounds an alarm when the mare sweats up in the first stage of labour. If the mare does not sweat, however, the alarm may not be triggered.

There are other systems for alerting you that your mare is in labour. In America these include devices that can be attached to the vulva or inserted inside the birth canal, which activate a transmitter when the mare starts to foal. The disadvantage with these systems is that the alarm only alerts you when labour has started, so you need to be nearby.

Much research has been done on testing the secretions of pre-foaling milk. It has been shown that there is an increase in calcium, magnesium and potassium and a reduction in the sodium content just prior to foaling. Various kits are available to test this. They are useful as a guide that the mare is or is not yet ready to foal, but the mare may still keep you waiting even when the electrolyte levels have changed.

Foaling

Most mares foal at night because they prefer to foal in a quiet environment. The first stage of labour may stop if they are disturbed. If you are watching a mare who is due to foal, be discreet and quiet so that she is not disturbed.

The birth is divided into three stages:

1 Increasing discomfort and colic-like pain due to the initial uterine contractions.
2 Rupture of the membranes, discharge of fluid and delivery of the foal. In the mare this is amazingly rapid and the foal should be delivered in an average of less than twenty minutes. Mares lie down for the delivery in 95 per cent of cases. If disturbed, a mare is more likely to stand up. If she keeps shifting her position it may suggest something is wrong and assistance should be sought. Normally the foal's front feet and then the head will rapidly appear, wrapped in the white membranes of the amniotic sac. One foot is usually slightly

A normal foaling: this is second stage labour and the foal's front legs can be seen emerging wrapped in the white membranes of the amniotic sac

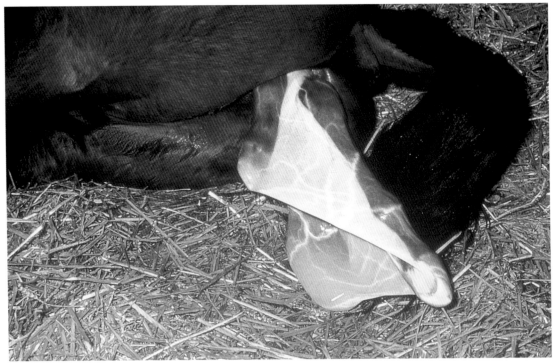

Gysbert van der Weijden DVM PhD

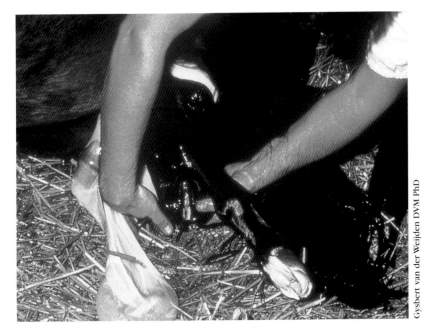

Assisting at a foaling: clearing the membranes so the foal can breathe

Gysbert van der Weijden DVM PhD

ahead of the other. This thick white membrane should rupture as the foal emerges, so that the foal can start to breathe. If a mare delivers in a standing position, assistance will be needed to catch the foal. Normally the mare will remain lying down for up to 40 minutes after delivery of her foal. It is perfectly natural that she should be allowed a chance to rest! (Owners are often concerned by the fact that she does not get up soon.) The umbilical cord remains intact after delivery of the foal. This cord links the foal to its supply system, the placenta. Immediately after delivery blood is still passing into the foal and a few minutes should be allowed to let this happen. It is important not to disturb the mare and foal at this stage. Try to allow the cord to break naturally as the mare and foal move. Providing the foal is breathing normally, allow the foal and its dam to get to know each other rather than interfere! If the cord does not break of its own accord, it can be cut and tied temporarily with sterile cord.

3   Delivery of the placenta. This should come away fairly quickly and the mare may show some discomfort as it is delivered. Once delivered it is important to check that it is intact and that no remnants are left within the mare.

If the placenta is still hanging from the vulva four to six hours after birth, it is described as a retained placenta and you should ring your vet for assistance.

Once the placenta has been passed it is best to save it in a bucket of water for your vet to examine. It is always sensible to ask your vet to check both mare and foal within 24 hours of the birth.

It is important that the placenta is checked after delivery to ensure that it is intact; if in doubt, ask your vet

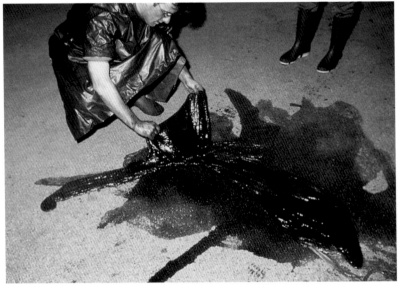

Gysbert van der Weijden DVM PhD

Complications of foaling

If the foal does not appear within twenty minutes of the mare lying down and straining hard, you will need immediate help from your vet.

For this reason, it is wise to alert your vet in advance that foaling is imminent. If your usual vet lives a long distance from where the mare is due to foal, ensure you have nearby veterinary assistance available as well.

In the rare case that a foal does become stuck, your vet may advise you to keep the mare up and walking round the box to reduce straining until help arrives. The action required will depend on individual circumstances. If the foal is wedged upside down, the mare may benefit from getting up and down to help reposition the foal. In other situations, the mare may only require gentle assistance to pull the foal into the world.

If the membranes that cover the foal do not break, human intervention may be needed to clear the foal's head so that it can breathe. You may simply need to cut the white bag (the amnion)

which is wrapped over the foal's head. In rare cases, the thickest part of the placenta (the chorion) will appear as a red velvety bulge rather than the normal white membranes. This is known as a 'red bag' and needs to be ruptured to allow safe passage of the foal.

Normally, when a mare foals the white membrane of the amniotic sac appears. In the case shown, the thickest part of the placenta is coming first. This is an emergency

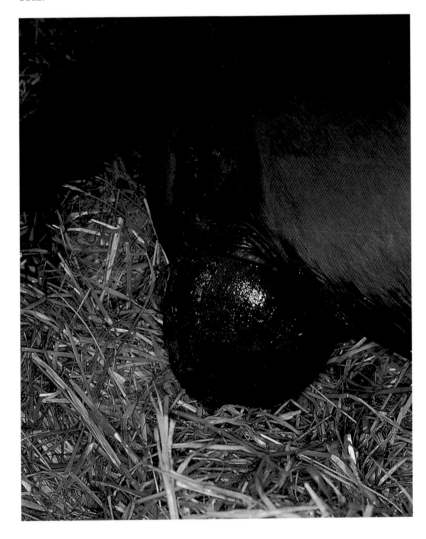

Always have available clean water and adequate help to assist the vet when he or she arrives at a foaling.

All of these problems appear daunting when written down but most are relatively straightforward once you have helped your first hundred mares to foal! If you do not have this experience, however, it is important to have experienced help available.

The newborn foal

The stress of foaling is more than compensated for by the arrival of a healthy foal. It is important to be aware that a foal is not a tiny 50 kg version of an adult horse, but a newborn baby adapting to life in the big wide world. The incredible thing is how quickly they do adapt compared to the human infant.

The normal healthy foal should stand within two hours and suck within four hours of birth.

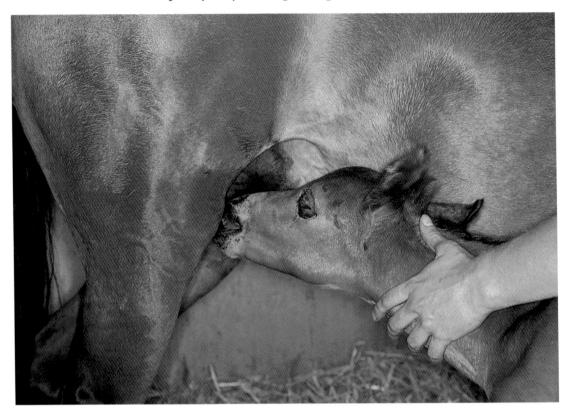

The foal should suckle from its dam as soon as possible after birth to absorb vital colostrum

A newborn foal should not be left more than six hours without a feed. Not only do they need the energy, but also, the first colostrum contains essential protection from infection for the foal. This is best obtained if the foal suckles from the dam within eight hours of birth. The majority of foals should nurse from their mother much sooner than that and the normal foal shows a suck reflex within twenty minutes of birth. Suckling is more effective than bottle-feeding or stomach tubing of colostrum.

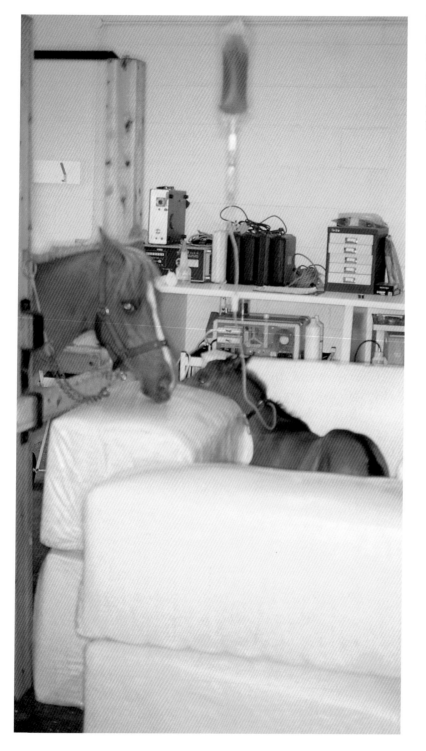

This foal failed to obtain enough antibodies from its dam's colostrum, so it is being given a transfusion of plasma to boost its immunity

If the mare runs milk steadily for more than twelve hours before foaling she may run out of colostrum for the foal. Your vet can do tests to check both the quality of the mare's colostrum and how effective the foal's colostrum uptake has been. It is vital that every foal has adequate colostrum. Without this protection against infection, a foal may not survive and all the effort of foaling may have been in vain!

The most important first aid treatments for a newborn foal are:

* to ensure it suckles from its dam
* to treat the fresh umbilical cord with an appropriate antiseptic, e.g. 0.5 per cent chorhexidine (Hibiscrub®) or tincture of iodine, which has a very effective drying action. Obtain whatever is most appropriate for your situation directly from your vet
* to watch the behaviour of the foal, ensure it bonds with the dam, feeds frequently, and passes urine and faeces. It is normal for foals to sleep a lot, like any other newborn, but it is important that they are alert and lively when they are awake
* either to ensure that the foal is given anti-tetanus treatment by your vet very soon after birth or, better still, ensure the dam is properly vaccinated in the last couple of months preceding foaling so that she can pass on this immunity to the foal.

A young foal is adapting to life in the big wide world and as it does so its pulse, breathing rate and temperature will change. It is important to recognise that a foal will differ in these respects to the normal rates for an adult horse.

Normal respiratory rate for a newborn foal at rest

Age	Respiratory rate (breaths per minute)
5 minutes	60–80
15 minutes	40–60
12 hours	30–40

Normal heart rate for a newborn foal at rest

Age	Heart rate (beats per minute)
Birth	60–80
0–2 hours	120–150
3 hours +	80–120
24 hours	80–100

Normal temperature for a newborn foal

If the temperature remains less than 99°F (37.2°C), help is needed to warm the foal with external heat, rugs, limb bandages, etc.

If the temperature is more than 102°F (38.8°C), help is needed to reduce external heat.

It will help if you can sit the foal up on its chest rather than leaving it to lie on its side. A foal that sits up will be better able to move air out of both its lungs. When carefully positioned sitting up, a sick foal is less at risk of developing pneumonia, damaging its underlying eye and other complications.

Foals are fragile creatures in their first few weeks of life. There is very little useful first aid advice that applies particularly to foals apart from WATCH them CLOSELY. Any change from the normal pattern of behaviour, particularly lethargy, sleeping more than usual and going 'off suck', i.e. failing to drink from their mother, should be taken seriously. Check the mare's udder to see if it is full. If you are in any doubt discuss your concerns with your vet. Examples of common foal problems include:

If a newborn foal is weak and cannot stand or suckle your vet should be contacted straightaway.

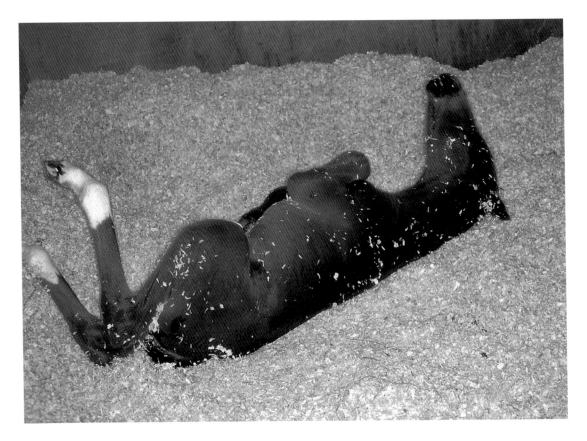

A foal with colic. A newborn can suffer from many unique problems in addition to facing the same problems as adult horses

Foal diarrhoea

Problems such as diarrhoea, which can be insignificant to an adult horse, are potentially life threatening in a foal. About 70 to 80 per cent of foals will have at least one episode of diarrhoea before they are six months old. Be aware that a foal will normally develop diarrhoea about six to fourteen days after it is born when its dam comes into season for the first time. This lasts two to four days and usually settles down without any treatment. The time to worry is if the diarrhoea persists, or the foal looks sick.

The only useful first aid treatment is to clean the foal's dirty rear end and apply petroleum jelly (Vaseline®) to protect the skin. If the diarrhoea does not dry up, veterinary help should be sought promptly.

Lameness in the foal

Any sign of lameness in the young foal should be taken seriously. A common cause for concern is infection within the joints of the foal, which has been shown to affect up to one per cent of Thoroughbred foals born each year. The signs to look out for are:

* suddenly obvious fairly severe lameness
* a degree of swelling and heat around the affected joint
* pain and reduced movement of the joint or joints involved
* a raised temperature.

Again, there is no magic first aid treatment. Instead, aggressive veterinary treatment will be needed. The best prevention is to ensure the foal has sufficient colostrum and that the umbilical cord is properly disinfected after birth.

Obviously there are other causes of lameness which also affect the foal. Another frequent cause for concern is when a foal is born with either bent or twisted legs, but many of these problems will rapidly improve as the foal grows. Until a foal with misshapen legs

Left: A young foal with an infection within the main joint of the hock which is bandaged. The neck is also bandaged to protect the catheter which is a tube inserted into the vein to inject frequent doses of antibiotics painlessly

Right: A close up of the same foal's infected hock. The area has been shaved to enable sterile surgery to drain the infection. Any foal with a swollen joint like this, and lameness, is a first aid emergency

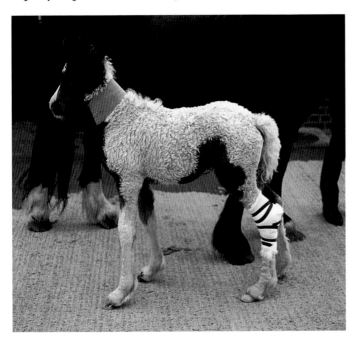

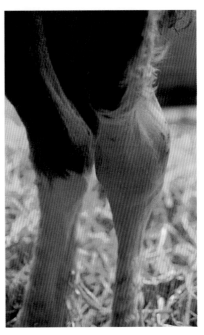

Any foal abnormality or illness should be taken as seriously, if not more so, than a similar condition in an adult horse.

is able to move well you should restrict its exercise. If you feel there is a significant problem, talk to your vet and your farrier.

Eye problems

Some foals are born with their eyelids turning inwards, so that the eyelashes rub on the eyeball. This is known as **entropion**. Initially, all you may notice is that the eye will be slightly runny or that there may be a mucky discharge. In these cases you should ask your vet to check the eyes promptly, as a minor corrective procedure can prevent permanent damage to the eye. Sometimes, this sort of eye problem is more likely to occur if a foal is weak and dehydrated, so it is important to look out for sore eyes in young foals.

Potential problems with the mare after foaling

Foal rejection

It cannot be overemphasised that it is vital that a foal should receive its first milk, i.e. colostrum, as soon as possible after birth. Occasionally, mares, particularly if they have not had a foal before, will reject their foal or not allow it to suckle. It will help if you have handled the mare's udder during her pregnancy so she is accustomed to something touching her teats in advance of the foal's arrival.

First aid with a mare who rejects her foal should include:

- ruling out medical conditions that cause a painful udder. Obviously, you may need to consult your vet
- trying to feed concentrates to the mare to distract her while the foal suckles
- asking your vet to check the mare and administer a sedative or tranquilliser to calm her. Avoid painful restraint of the mare, if possible, as it will only stress her more
- a final approach, although more dangerous, is to turn the mare and foal out with other mares and foals in an attempt to

114

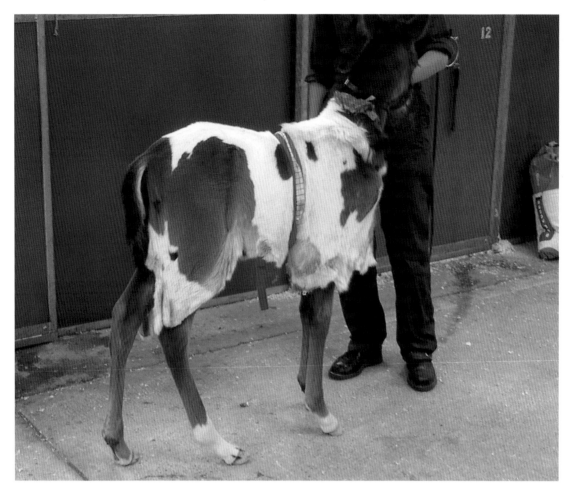

encourage maternal behaviour in the mare. If you do this, however, you need to observe the group closely all the time.

If treatment is not successful, you may end up milking the mare and feeding the foal its colostrum by bottle or stomach tube. If the mare will not accept the foal or if she dies at birth, you may be left with no alternative except to rear the foal as an orphan or, better still, find a foster mother for it. Foals need other horses for company and those that are hand reared can become difficult to handle later on. In the UK there is a National Foaling Bank (Tel: 01952 811234, Fax: 01952 811202) which can often provide extremely useful advice and assistance in these circumstances, as can your own veterinary surgeon.

An orphan foal wearing the skin of the mare's own dead foal like a rug to persuade the mare to accept the strange foal

Mastitis

This is infection of the udder and is unusual in the mare as compared to other animals. It can be found in lactating mares, but also within eight weeks of weaning.

What to look for:

- a swollen udder, which may only involve one side of the udder
- pain if the udder is touched
- swelling along the lower abdomen, i.e. **ventral oedema**
- fever
- depression
- loss of appetite.

The vet should be contacted and a visit is usually required within 24 hours, particularly if the foal is still with the mare. If the mare will allow it, it is usually best if the foal can continue to feed. In the majority of cases the foal will be unaffected by the infection and removing milk from the udder will help the mare. In some cases, however, the mare will not permit the foal to feed, if the foal is young or weak, you should check with your own vet. The majority of cases occur after weaning when the foal is not a problem. Most cases respond very well to rapid treatment.

Pelvic fractures

Pelvic fractures can occur after a difficult foaling, especially if excessive force was used to remove the foal. Another cause is a heavy fall during foaling, following loss of balance or a collapse through pain. The mare will be lame and may be unable to stand. The vet should be called if the mare still cannot stand more than two hours after foaling. For this reason foaling boxes should have non-slip floors to reduce the risk of a mare 'doing the splits'.

Post-foaling colic

Many mares will look a little uncomfortable after foaling. Mild discomfort in the mare is normal after foaling but should reduce within one to two hours. Frequently, this is associated with bruising from the trauma of foaling and/or the contractions of the uterus, particularly when the foal first starts to feed. It can be hard to be certain if the pain originates from the uterus or the bowel. In fact, there are a variety of different causes of colic pain in a mare after foaling, some of which are potentially serious. The list of possible problems include:

- a rupture of the uterus
- internal bleeding
- bowel bruising, tears or ruptures.

All of these are unusual, however it is best to rule them out by a careful veterinary examination. Basically, if a mare is becoming increasingly uncomfortable after foaling, you should contact your vet to discuss the signs shown. You may well require an emergency visit. If a mare's post-foaling colic pains do not subside following a ten-minute walk (always walk her around close to and within sight of the foal), then you should talk to your vet.

Much more common is an impactive colic, where the mare fails to pass droppings after foaling, often because she is sore and uncomfortable. This can be helped by a laxative diet, i.e. bran mashes, and light exercise, i.e. turn out in a paddock. Your vet may be needed to administer drugs such as liquid paraffin.

Post-foaling bleeding (haemorrhage)

The normal mare will discharge some blood from the vagina after foaling. This may increase in amount four or five days after foaling as the mare starts to come into season, i.e. the 'foaling heat'. This is perfectly normal and not a cause for concern. The time to worry is if the bleeding becomes profuse (i.e. more than

If a mare has a discharge as shown, she should be watched and your vet consulted in case she has a uterine infection (metritis)

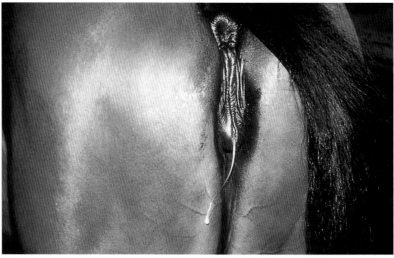

Dr Paul J de Vries DVM

If a pregnant or recently foaled mare shows signs of unusually severe colic, pale mucous membranes and a weak rapid pulse, internal bleeding must be suspected. This is an emergency and your vet should be contacted straightaway.

a large dribble) or if it turns an unpleasant colour so that it is more like watery pus. This would suggest an internal infection of the uterus known as **metritis**. This requires veterinary treatment, not as an immediate emergency but within the next 24 to 36 hours. Certainly, if you are intending to breed from the mare, it is sensible to control any such infections promptly. If left untreated the mare is more at risk from complications, particularly laminitis, especially in the heavier breeds of horse.

Internal bleeding after foaling is a much more serious problem. This is more common in older mares who have had several foals previously. It can occur before foaling or any time from 30 minutes to several weeks after foaling. The early signs may be masked by normal post-foaling discomfort. Unfortunately there is often little that can be done apart from pain control and supportive measures to help control major internal bleeding. Even so, you should still call the vet to confirm the diagnosis and control the pain.

Retained placenta

A retained placenta is when a mare has not delivered the afterbirth within four to six hours of foaling. During most normal foalings, the placenta and foetal membranes that sur-

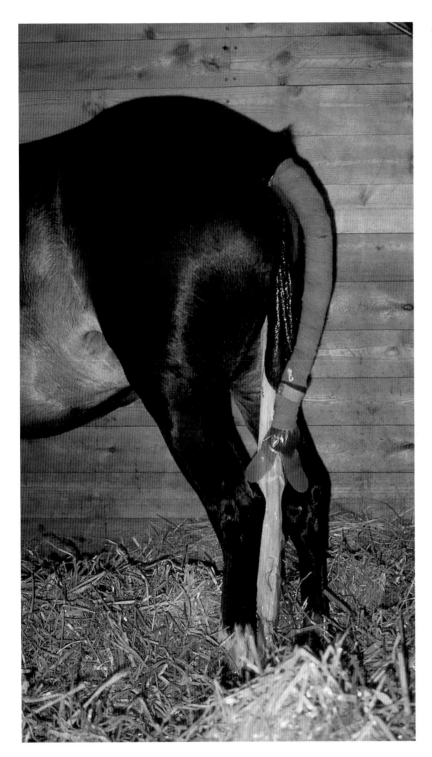

A retained placenta in a mare

rounded and protected the foal inside the mare are delivered soon after the foal. In fact, somewhere between two and ten per cent of mares will fail to pass their placenta within three hours from foaling. If a mare retains her placenta for more than four hours, it is time to be concerned and contact your vet. If nothing has happened after six hours, it should be considered as a potentially life-threatening emergency. A retained placenta provides a wide open door for infection to get inside the mare and cause serious complications. The mare is likely to be less fertile, particularly if attempts are made to breed at the foaling heat, which usually occurs seven to ten days after foaling.

How do you know your mare has a retained placenta

- If the placenta can be seen dangling from the back end of the mare, the problem is obvious.
- The placenta may tear and part may remain concealed internally. It is therefore a good idea to examine the membranes after delivery to ensure that nothing is missing. The placenta is approximately Y-shaped, with the membranes attached to it. There will be at least one obvious hole in it, through which the foal exited. Other tears may be due to the mare standing on it, so it should be pieced together like a jigsaw.
- Occasionally the placenta is not visible, as the foetal membranes may have slipped forward and remain inside the mare. An unusually dirty discharge may suggest this.
- If a mare becomes ill within a couple of days of foaling, with a high temperature, loss of appetite, depression and laminitis, a fragment of retained placenta should be suspected and the vet contacted straightaway.

What you should do if you think the placenta is retained

- If there is any reason for concern, i.e. the placenta is retained for more than three hours, you must contact your vet. Some mares will remain relatively well with a retained placenta, whilst others can die from it. It is a more dangerous condition in heavy horse breeds. One of the reasons for this is that laminitis can be a complication. This can have dire consequences for breeds such as Shires. The rule is, the bigger the horse, the more serious the problem, and the more urgently treatment should be initiated.

- If the membranes are dangling, it can help to tie a knot in them above the hocks. This will prevent the mare from treading on them, as well as keeping them cleaner. However, some mares are alarmed by the feel of the dangling placenta against their legs.
- It is *not* recommended to tie a weight to the placenta to encourage it to be expelled as this may cause internal tearing and bleeding.
- For the same reason, it is not generally considered a good idea to pull out the dangling placenta. A gentle tug, as if shaking hands with someone, is worth trying in case it has detached and is just sitting within the uterus, but no excessive force should be applied.
- Encouraging the foal to suckle will produce a natural response in the mare which will help to expel the placenta.
- Gentle exercise, e.g. a five-minute walk, may help shift the placenta.

What will your vet do?

This will depend on the individual case. The majority of cases will respond to injections of oxytocin which stimulates contractions of the uterus (i.e. womb) and pushes out the placenta. Such drugs are often given in the form of an intravenous drip. Occasionally the vet will need to distend the placenta with fluid to encourage it to be expelled. Antibiotic and anti-inflammatory drugs are also often prescribed, together with measures to reduce the risk of laminitis.

If treated within hours, it is likely there will be no long lasting ill effects for either mare or foal. Cattle can cope for days with a retained placenta without major problems; horses are more delicate creatures and require rapid treatment.

Uterine prolapse

Uterine prolapse is when the uterus is passed out through the vagina. This is a very rare emergency that can happen in the 24 hours after foaling. If it does it is obvious as an enormous thick red corrugated mass hanging from the mare's back end. It should not be confused with the normal placenta being passed, which is much thinner and darker in colour.

If this happens you should call your vet immediately, requesting an emergency visit as soon as possible.

What you should do whilst waiting for the vet to arrive

1 Try to keep the mare standing still pending the vet's arrival. This is to prevent the mare causing damage to the uterus or pushing more of it out.
2 A large warm wet towel or sheet may be wrapped around the organ to protect and support it. If the mare is quiet, it will help to hold the prolapse up on a sheet to reduce swelling or any further damage.
3 Make sure you have towels, sheets and clean water ready for the vet. Sometimes the vet may apply sugar to the prolapse to help reduce the swelling, so, if practical, have a couple of bags of ordinary kitchen sugar handy.

What will the vet do?

The vet will treat a uterine prolapse by giving the mare drugs to reduce any straining and then gently clean and replace the prolapse.

Once the uterus has been put back, the mare will be stitched and given further drugs to prevent it happening again. The prognosis for future breeding is good if the replacement is straightforward and the problem will not necessarily happen again at future foalings. Unfortunately, things can go wrong before the placenta is replaced. The tissues may tear, resulting in a fatal haemorrhage or a prolapse of the bowel. Sometimes the mare may succumb to shock.

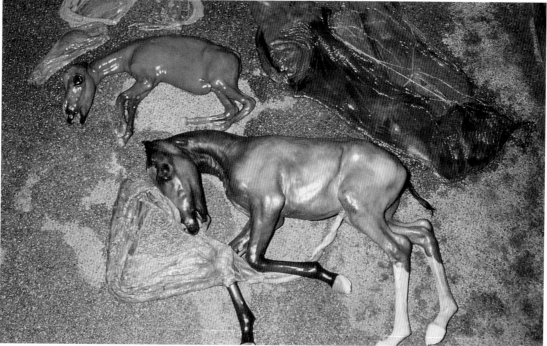

Herman Jonker DVM PhD

Potential pre-foaling problems

Abortion

Between ten and fifteen per cent of pregnant mares do not carry their foals to term. Abortion is defined as the loss of the foal and its membranes before the three-hundreth (300) day of gestation. This can happen for all sorts of different reasons, even when the mare has been looked after immaculately. Frequently there are no warning signs and one simply finds the dead foal. On other occasions the aborted foal is not even discovered and the mare is simply found to be no longer pregnant when checked at a later date.

When a mare does abort, she may seem remarkably well, but it is sensible to ring your vet straightaway to arrange for her to be checked and to examine the dead foal to find out why this has happened. If other pregnant mares are in contact with the one that has aborted it should be considered an emergency. This is because of a virus (**equine herpes virus**) which is infectious and

Before the use of ultrasound scanning to help detect twins in the early stages of pregnancy, twins (as shown here) were the commonest cause of abortion in the mare

can cause multiple abortions within a group of mares. For this reason, following an abortion it is sensible to:

- contact the vet straightaway
- isolate the mare in a stable
- put the aborted foal and membranes in a leak-proof container
- disinfect the area where the abortion occurred, e.g. with Virkon®.

There is a detailed code of practice, drawn up by the Thoroughbred Breeders Association, which gives useful guidance as to what to do to minimise the spread of infectious reproductive diseases, particularly viral abortion. It can be obtained from:

- The British Horse Society, Welfare Department, British Equestrian Centre, Stoneleigh Park, Kenilworth, Warwickshire CV8 2LR. Tel: 01203 696697
- The Horserace Betting Levy Board (HRBLB), 52 Grovenor Gardens, London SW1W OAU. Tel: 0207 333 0043
- The Thoroughbred Breeders Association, Stanstead House, The Avenue, Newmarket, Suffolk CB8 9AA. Tel: 01638 661321.

Abdominal or ventral swelling

It is normal for many pregnant mares to develop a certain amount of soft swelling or **oedema** (i.e. fluid swelling under the skin which reduces if you press it) around and in front of the udder. Occasionally they may move stiffly as a result of this. Treatment is usually not required, apart from light exercise, e.g. turn them out to graze.

Occasionally pregnant mares will develop enormous abdominal swellings which may be a consequence of fluid accumulation internally, known as **hydrops of the placental membranes**, when the mare will have an enormously round distended abdomen. Other serious abdominal swellings are **rupture of the ventral abdominal muscles** and or the **prepubic tendon**. In such cases the abdomen bulges underneath and the swelling does not go down with exercise. There is no first aid treatment to manage

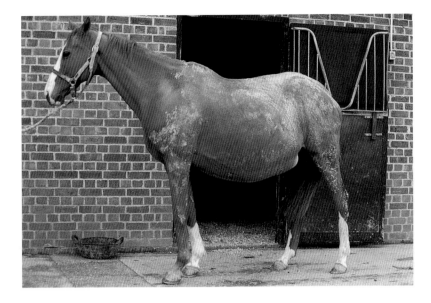

Many heavily pregnant mares will develop a soft fluid swelling underneath their belly. This is ventral oedema

this, but it is best to consult your vet to assess the significance of any abdominal swelling that does not reduce with exercise.

Gestational length

The average length of gestation in the mare is 342 days, but it can easily range from 320 to 365 days. Some mares have been known to carry their foal for even longer with minimal ill effects.

Foals which are born a month before their so-called due date are likely to be weak and will require intensive nursing to survive. If they are much more premature than a month they have virtually no chance of survival. It may be kinder to put a very premature foal to sleep rather than struggle for days and nights for the same eventual outcome. This is something to discuss with your own vet at the time, depending on the individual circumstances of the case.

Prolonged gestation is common in the mare and is not necessarily an indication of any problem. Mares have been recorded to have pregnancies lasting thirteen months. It is not like people where induction is necessary if a mother is slightly overdue. In the mare it is best to wait until she is ready to foal, unless there is a very good reason to do otherwise. Again, you should be guided by your veterinary surgeon.

Never expect your mare to foal the day she is due!

125

Pre-foaling colic

In the later stages of pregnancy mares can develop a variety of different colic problems. Some involve the uterus and unborn foal directly, whilst others are a gastrointestinal problem, often complicated by the amount of space occupied by the growing foal within the mare's abdomen. Colic may also be an indication of impending abortion, so it should be taken seriously because of the risk to the unborn foal. If your pregnant mare has colic, you should contact your vet for advice. Many mares can develop impactions late on in pregnancy and it is advisable to reduce the chance of this happening by feeding a relatively laxative diet, e.g. regular bran mashes.

Running milk

Mares may run milk prior to foaling. This is not detrimental to the mare in itself, but can be an indication of abortion or premature delivery. The condition itself should not be treated but the mare should be watched carefully for any underlying disorder. If a mare runs milk just before she is due to foal, she may lose all the vital colostrum that she should pass to the foal. In such cases a blood sample should be taken from the foal at around 24 hours of age to ensure it has sufficient immunity. If a foal has not received sufficient immunity, a transfusion of plasma may be required as an emergency measure to provide the vital protective antibodies.

Plasma for transfusion can be obtained by taking blood from another horse and removing the red cells by spinning the blood and collecting the antibody-rich plasma, or else a commercially available antibody-rich plasma can be used. The commercial plasma bags can be stored frozen so that they are always readily available. Newborn foals who have not received adequate colostrum usually require approximately 1–2 litres of plasma to improve their antibody status but follow up blood tests should be performed to check this. If the foal is already sick, a larger volume of plasma may be necessary.

Stallion first aid

Injuries to the penis

The stallion is very vulnerable to trauma when he attempts to cover an uncooperative mare. If kicked (particularly when erect) the penis may swell rapidly as a result of bleeding within the internal structures. Any wound to the penis is liable to bleed profusely and immediate first aid should include:

- removal of the mare and attempting to calm the stallion
- application of cold water, either by hose or by application of wet towels
- support of the penis and prepuce is very important to avoid further damage as the weight of the damaged tissue will pull it downwards and make the injury worse. In an emergency it is possible to make a very effective truss from old tights, which will permit urination without retaining moisture or chafing

Fitting a truss to support an injury to the penis caused by the stallion attempting to jump over a stable door and becoming stuck halfway

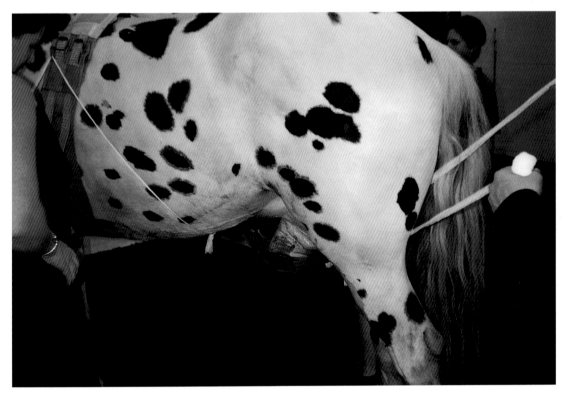

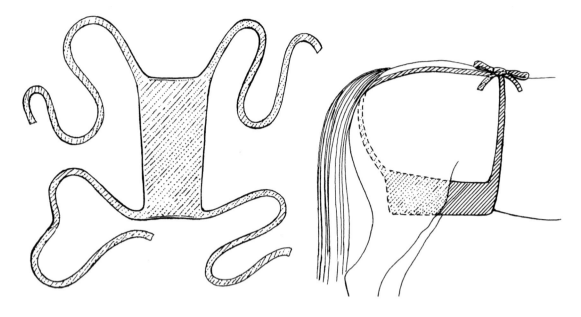

Support of the penis within the sheath is important when the area is injured. A support can be made as shown. Two pairs of tights sewn together at the top will work well for this

the skin. Your vet should be contacted before you attempt to fit such a device. However, in case they might be needed, it may be worth ensuring that you have two pairs of old tights available!

Your vet should be called immediately in this sort of emergency. The stallion will need pain-killing drugs and other essential treatment as soon as possible.

Testicular trauma

The scrotum is also relatively vulnerable to kick injuries. The damage may result in a permanent reduction in fertility unless prompt and effective treatment is undertaken. Again first aid should include cold hosing or application of wet towels. Although cold water is a useful first aid treatment, it must not be overused here, as too much cold water treatment can make the delicate skin soggy and damage the tissues. Again, your vet should be consulted as an immediate emergency. In some cases your vet may elect to remove the compromised testicle to prevent damage to the other one from inflammation.

Enlarged testicles

The testicles may become swollen after an injury such as a kick, but other potential problems include:

- an infection in one or both testicles, known as **orchitis**
- a **hernia**, where a section of bowel escapes from the abdomen into the scrotum. This may be a cause of colic in entire animals
- a twisted testicle, i.e. **testicular torsion**, which, again, can be a rare cause of colic
- a tumour.

Rather than using any first aid remedies, it is advisable to contact your vet. If the horse appears to be in pain or there is a concern relating to fertility, an emergency visit may be needed.

> *There are many potential problems associated with breeding horses. It is not something to undertake lightly!*

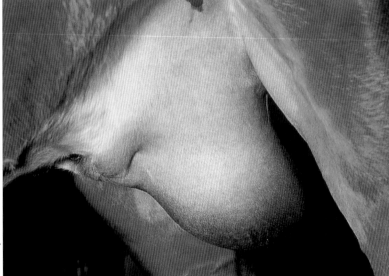

Herman Jonker DVM PhD

A stallion with a swollen testicle like this one requires urgent veterinary attention. In this case a severe infection was present, known as orchitis, and emergency veterinary attention was needed

7. MAJOR DISASTERS: PREVENTION, PLANNING AND AVOIDANCE

Tetanus

Every year equine vets see the occasional case of tetanus, and of the cases diagnosed, very few will survive. The tragedy is that this is a disease that is very easily prevented by a safe, effective and inexpensive vaccination that is readily available. Everybody should know about this life-threatening disease which can affect both you and your horses!

Tetanus is caused by bacteria which normally live in the soil but which can enter the body of either a person or a horse, usually through a wound. Dirty wounds which are not exposed to fresh air are the highest risk; in particular, deep penetrating wounds such as nail punctures in the foot. Having said that, tetanus bacteria can attack via the tiniest graze, and I have seen tetanus develop from the gaps in the gum around a loose tooth in a youngster. Horses and ponies are the most susceptible domestic animal species. Dogs very rarely develop tetanus and so are not routinely vaccinated.

The disease of tetanus is caused by the release of poison (known as toxin) by the bacteria. This toxin is deadly and will spread through the body, affecting the nervous system. Tetanus cases are seen much more rarely now that an effective vaccine is available, but they still do happen. Unfortunately, because the disease is now rare, due to vaccination, people forget to have their horses injected and then the disease starts to reappear. If you ever saw a case you would make certain that both you and your animals were fully protected by regular vaccination. The vaccine is very safe, it does not cost a lot, and there is really no excuse for not using it.

The illness caused by tetanus is commonly known as **lockjaw**. This is because in the later stages of the disease the horse's mouth clamps shut so that the animal cannot eat or drink. In the early stages of the disease the signs to look for are:

- general stiffness, especially a rigid, stiff neck
- colic in the early stages
- high temperature
- the top of the tail sticking out, and the ears sticking up
- stiff tense legs so that the horse looks like a toy rocking horse
- standing immobile with a grimacing expression and flared nostrils
- general muscle spasms
- membranes of the eye extending over the eyeball, particularly if the head is lifted.

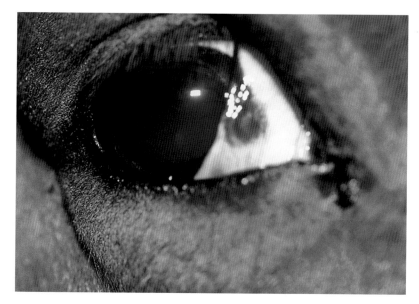

The membrane (or third eyelid) is extending over the eyeball. This is a sign of tetanus

In many cases of tetanus the wound where the germ entered is never found. So do not wait till a horse cuts himself before you have him vaccinated. Make sure all your horses and ponies are vaccinated regularly against tetanus.

Make sure you are also vaccinated against tetanus and not just your horses.

If you see any suspicion signs, call your vet straightaway. Frequently there is no obvious wound to explain how the disease started, so-called '**idiopathic tetanus**'. It is a very serious disease which can cause a lot of suffering. Even with intensive treatment, about three-quarters of tetanus cases die. Those that do survive are those cases that were caught early and have intensive and expensive treatment. The rule of thumb I use is that if a tetanus case is unable to stand, it is actually kindest if it is destroyed immediately since the chance of recovery is remote. A recent survey showed that all the cases that were recumbent when diagnosed did not survive. Those that did recover required lengthy periods of intensive veterinary care and diligent nursing. If a horse survives a case of tetanus, it will not develop immunity. Vaccination is always essential.

If you buy a new pony and you are uncertain if he has been vaccinated before, it is best to start the vaccination course again. The primary vaccination course consists of two doses of **tetanus toxoid** vaccine, which are given by intramuscular injection four to six weeks apart. A booster injection is required a year later, and after that you should ask your vet how often you need to get it done. Tetanus is more common in certain areas of the UK where it may be advisable to have more regular boosters. Keep a record of all tetanus inoculations.

If an unvaccinated horse or pony is injured, it will be at risk of catching tetanus, so it is normal to treat them with **tetanus antitoxin**. This will act quickly to fight the disease by neutralising any tetanus toxins present at that time, but it is no substitute for proper vaccination. The problem with this tetanus antitoxin is that it does not last, so it is important to start the vaccination programme as well. The tetanus antitoxin is an antiserum which can also be used to treat horses with the disease. In severe tetanus cases it may even be injected into the linings around the brain in a desperate measure to save a life. Antibiotics, muscle relaxants, painkillers and sedatives are also used as treatment, but prevention is best of all.

Fires and burns

A fire in a barn full of horses has to be one's worst nightmare. Recent American work has estimated that faulty electrical wiring causes 80 per cent of fires in agricultural buildings. The chance of a fire is said to be greater in a building that is more than five years old. Many of the places where we stable our horses are potential firetraps and it is sensible to look at the problem and have a plan ready before there is a crisis.

A fire involving combustible materials (wood, straw, hay, shavings, etc.) doubles in size every minute. Therefore in ten minutes a fire will increase in size by more than 4,000 times.

What to consider

- How would you get the horses out in an emergency? Does the barn have more than one exit? This is a big safety advantage of double-ended American style barns.
- If you open the doors to let the horses escape, where will they go? If the yard gate is open for the Fire Brigade, you need to ensure the horses can be driven out into a field. Further accidents can happen if the horses escape onto the road which may be partially obscured by smoke.
- Do you have fire extinguishers available and do you know how to use them?
- Do people smoke around the stables? All stable yards should have a no smoking policy!
- Are there any emergency lights? Smoke from a fire will obscure everything.
- What would your horse do if he met a fireman dressed up in all his kit?
- Do you ever have a fire drill? It is sensible to practise horse evacuation before a crisis.
- Is there an instruction sheet on what to do if there is a fire?
- Is there any fire detection equipment or fire extinguishers?
- Is there room between barns for fire engines to get close enough to work.
- Is there room to evacuate horses? Keep the barn clear of clutter, especially inflammable materials such as hay and straw.
- Is there a headcollar and lead rope by every box, so that you can quickly lead a horse out of the way of danger? In a fire,

leather headcollars are safer as nylon ones will melt with the heat. For the same reason wooden latches on doors are recommended, as metal ones can become too hot to touch in a fire.

- All light bulbs should have a metal cage around them, not to keep the horse away from the glass, but to avoid hay, straw or shavings landing on a hot bulb and catching fire.
- Is there a hose all ready attached to a tap? Water is an effective extinguisher of fires in hay, straw and shavings. Electrical or flammable liquid fires require a chemical fire extinguisher.
- Are there towels to hand? In an emergency, could these be soaked with water to cover the eyes and nose of a horse to help lead it away from the fire without panicking?

In the majority of cases, these questions are not ever answered until a crisis occurs. Fortunately, most people are well enough aware of the risks of fire and so are careful around horses. Having said that, a stable fire can be such an enormous disaster that it is well worth some advance planning. Your local fire station may be able to give you further advice.

What to do if there is a fire

1 Shout for help and sound the fire alarm.
2 Call the Fire Brigade.
3 Try to extinguish the fire.
4 First ensure human safety, then help the horses.
5 Block horse access to the roads. The instinctive thing to do is just open the stable doors and let the horses out. It is vital they are directed away from further danger, e.g. into an enclosed field and not out on the road to collide with the Fire Brigade. It is worth having a practice!

If you cannot get a horse out, blindfold him with any wet cloth that is to hand, also pulling it down over the nostrils to reduce the smell of the fire. Horses may be too terrified to leave their stable and, unfortunately, if you cannot get them out, you must consider your own safety first.

First aid for horses affected by a fire

In a stable fire, horses may be seriously affected by, or may even die from smoke inhalation. They can die without actual skin burns.

Horses suffering from smoke inhalation will be breathless and coughing. Ideally you should get them into an area of fresh air away from the smoke, where they can stand quietly away from all the fuss associated with a fire.

Skin burns are not always as bad as they look, depending on how deep they are. Skin typically takes a long time to absorb heat, so the longer the individual has been exposed, the worse the situation will be.

Immediate first aid for a skin burn is to cool the affected area (use ice or cold water) to draw out heat and reduce further damage. Hosing the area of damage for at least ten minutes is another useful way of doing this.

At the same time, horses caught in or near a fire will be frightened and very shocked, so good supportive care is essential.

You should contact your vet straightaway requesting an immediate emergency visit. If there is traffic congestion as a result of the fire, ensure the vet can get through to the area where the horses are.

Transport

There are many occasions when a horse will need to be transported from the scene of an initial accident or injury. This may just be for a short distance, for instance, back to the stable yard near the course of an event. Longer distance transport may be required to an appropriate equine veterinary clinic with facilities to cope with major emergencies, e.g. if it is thought that a horse may be suffering from a twisted gut which may require surgery.

There are many occasions when it is sensible to move a horse to a place with better facilities to provide adequate first aid. Many vets would prefer a sick or injured horse to come to their own veterinary clinic where specialised equipment is available, e.g. an X-ray machine to diagnose and treat the horse most effectively.

What is best for each horse will need to be decided on the basis of the individual circumstances at the time. At the end of the day only the veterinary surgeon is qualified to decide whether an injured horse is fit to travel. There will be situations where it is inhumane to travel an injured horse and it may be kinder to have the horse destroyed where the accident has happened, rather than prolong his ordeal.

On the other hand, in many cases, moving a horse is the only way of ensuring effective first aid, good follow-up treatment and a full recovery; hence there is a need to travel sick and injured horses. An injured or sick horse can travel in normal horse transport provided there is sufficient space for him to be comfortable and the loading and unloading set-up is safe. If a horse has a leg injury, it is particularly important that the lorry or trailer ramp does not have a steep slope and it is ideal if proper loading and unloading ramps can be used. There is evidence that horses travel better facing backwards but this will depend on what is possible in the transport available. There is also an argument for the horse travelling with the lame limb nearest the rear of the vehicle, so that it can cope better with braking forces. In some situations, you may be advised to leave the head untied or on a long rope to allow the horse to balance better. Whatever way the horse is positioned in a box or transport, it is important to consider ease of unloading.

Special equine ambulance trailers are available. It is obligatory to have them at all racecourse meetings. The Jockey Club approved ambulance has to have the following:

- a low-loading capability with long, shallow, sloped front and rear ramps
- internal, moveable padded partitions
- a belly sling to help support an unsteady horse
- adequate headroom
- internal lighting
- a means of communicating with the driver.

Equally important are adequate ventilation, well-inflated tyres and good suspension to provide a smooth and comfortable ride.

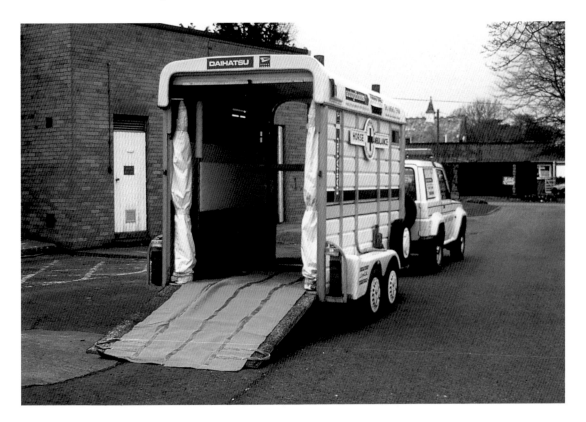

For the same reason a good driver is an absolute essential, prob- ably more important than anything else. Many horses feel much more relaxed in their own familiar box.

Horses are safer if they are travelled in appropriate protective clothing, e.g. travelling boots, poll guard (see page 45). In an emergency, however, when a horse needs to be moved rapidly, it is better to travel without these things rather than wait for the appropriate gear to be found.

You should consult your vet as to whether an ill or injured horse requires painkillers to travel. In many cases the horse will relax more with a good support bandage (if needed) and a hay net, rather than medication. Painkillers or sedatives may result in further injury as the horse may become unaware of the original problem and make it worse, e.g. by putting too much weight on an injured leg. Sedation may make a horse wobbly and less safe to travel. Again it will depend on individual circumstances.

The best first aid advice is to ensure that you have good and

Purpose-designed equine ambulances may be available at major competitions to permit the safe transport of injured horses. Note the low ramp and drag sheet for shifting a horse if necessary

reliable horse transport and a capable driver available for the time when they may be needed, even in the middle of the night in midwinter!

Euthanasia

Having your horse or pony put down is probably the worst first aid emergency that a horse owner has to face with their own animal. It is appropriate to consider this as part of first aid, since, unfortunately, there are emergencies where it is the only humane solution. Certainly, it is far kinder than allowing an animal with an irreparable injury to continue suffering. It is best to think ahead as in an emergency you may be asked to make an immediate decision. For your horse's sake, it is best to consider the possibility in advance.

In an emergency situation of such severity, the vet will have been called and will advise you what the options are and what is best for your horse's welfare. If the horse has to be put down, the vet will advise you on how this is to be done. Basically, either a lethal injection or a gun may be used to put the horse down as quickly and humanely as possible.

It is worth remembering that euthanasia literally means 'a good death' and that is what one aims to achieve. A very clear and sympathetic booklet is produced by the Humane Slaughter Association (see address on page 154).

Notification

If the horse is insured, the insurance company must be told that you are considering having your horse put down. You should obtain their agreement to proceed in advance, if it is at all practical to do so. In a major emergency, of course, e.g. a horse with a broken leg, then it is reasonable to have the horse put down first and tell the insurers as soon as possible afterwards.

It is ideal, although not always possible, to tell insurers before a horse is actually destroyed. Insurance companies may well request that a vet perform an examination of the horse after death, so you must allow this to happen, if required.

Disposal

This may be taken out of your hands if an accident happens in a public area. The arrangements vary in different areas. However, the options usually include:

- the carcass being collected by the local knackerman or huntsman
- animal cremation, where you can arrange to have the ashes returned to you. There is a limited availability for this and the charges can be high
- incineration, which is a more economic, similar option, but you are unable to have any ashes back
- burial is permitted in certain sites. You are obliged to obtain permission from the National Rivers Authority and the local Environmental Health Department.

If the horse has had medication administered, the carcass is unlikely to be suitable for feeding, e.g. to hounds. Alternative arrangements may need to be made. This should be checked with the vet and huntsman/knackerman involved.

Insurance

If you own a horse, it is a sensible precaution to have adequate insurance cover. Unlike cars, this is not a legal requirement, however it would be foolish not even to take out public liability cover. It is obviously possible to have far more comprehensive insurance cover to protect you and your horse against death, accident, injury, illness and medical/veterinary fees, plus a variety of other potential risks. Usually, the more comprehensive the cover, the higher the premium. The many alternatives offered by the different companies are widely advertised. If you do decide to insure your horse it is sensible to ask your vet which company he or she recommends. The recommended companies can then advise you on the different policies that are available. Always inform your insurers as soon as your horse is ill or injured, keeping a clear record of all the details.

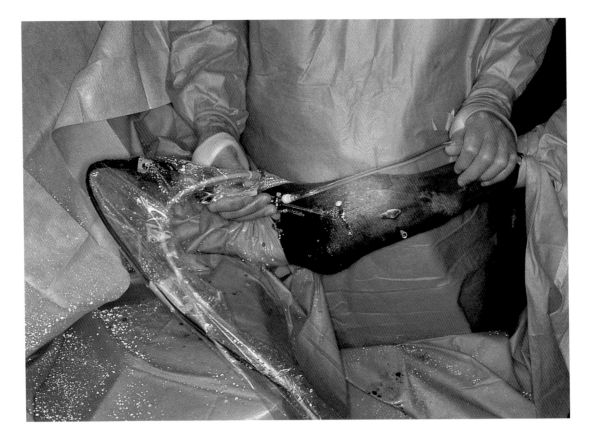

Surgery in the horse can be complex and costly. This should be considered when thinking about insurance cover. For instance, this shows a horse's infected hock joint undergoing flushing with sterile saline to clean it and arthroscopic examination (looking inside the joint with a tiny telescope-like instrument) to assess the degree of damage after a small wound penetrated a joint

Permanent incapacity (or permanent loss of use [i.e. PLOU]) cover

This means that insurers will agree to pay the sum insured for a horse that becomes permanently and totally incapable of doing whatever it was insured to do, e.g. show jump. Such a claim will only be met if all reasonable treatment options have been tried and failed, plus the horse has been given sufficient time to recover and still can no longer do whatever is required of him. This can enable horses to remain in retirement when they are no longer capable of working, for instance a horse with navicular disease that can do light hacking but will never show jump again. Frequently, insurers will require that such horses are freeze branded to denote the horse is the subject of a previously settled insurance claim.

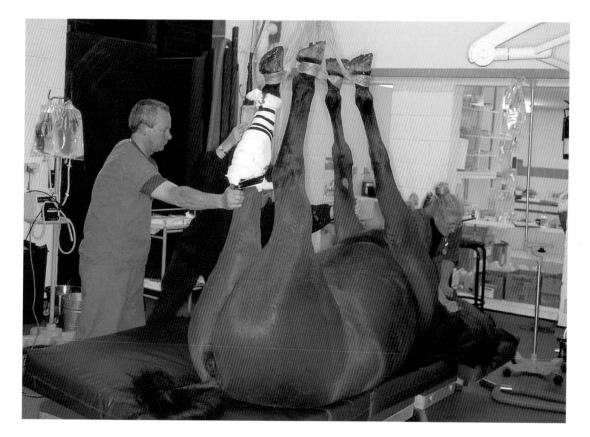

Humane destruction (or all risks mortality [i.e. ARM] or death) cover

This is a much more limited insurance cover, which normally means that your insurers will only pay out if the horse actually dies or has to be put down on humane grounds. This really means restricted insurance cover. It will only pay out if the insured horse sustains an injury or manifests an illness or disease that is so severe as to warrant immediate destruction to relieve incurable and excessive pain and that no other options are available to that horse at that time. This can lead to confusion in that it means this sort of insurance cover will permit a claim for the horse which has a irreparable fracture, but not the horse that has sustained a tendon injury. The tendon injury might initially seem just as painful, yet if treated properly, long term, the tendon

This horse is being moved into the operating theatre under general anaesthesia in preparation for surgery on a leg

141

This is a post-mortem picture of a horse that had severe colic associated with the overwhelming number of worms (ascarids) it carried within its bowel. It had not been regularly wormed

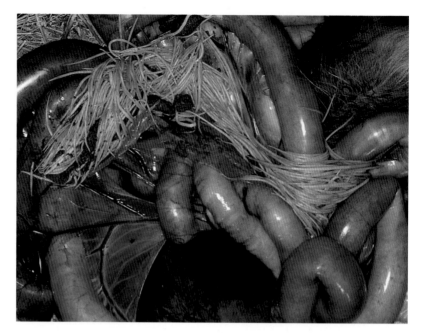

Remember that prevention of problems does not only involve major issues like insurance and fire precautions, but also the routine management of your horse and pony. It is essential to take proper care of day to day matters, such as frequent worm control measures, regular footcare and vaccinations.

injury case would become sound enough to potter round the paddock. On the same basis, cases of navicular disease will usually be able to cope at grass but are unable to work hard. Such cases would be likely to meet the requirements of a permanent incapacity policy but not a humane destruction policy.

How much veterinary fees cover does your insurance policy have?

It is wise to check the level of cover involved for any one incident. Surgery, for instance for colic, can amount to several thousand pounds. Some policies will provide cover of only a few hundred pounds per incident, which is inadequate. Most policies will also expect you to pay an excess, e.g. the first £100 of any claim for veterinary fees. This should be checked, as should any exclusions or other restrictions *before* there is an emergency and it is too late.

As far as your horse is concerned, modern veterinary diagnosis and treatments are becoming more sophisticated and hence more costly all the time. Think now whether it would be right to submit your horse to costly treatment and whether you could

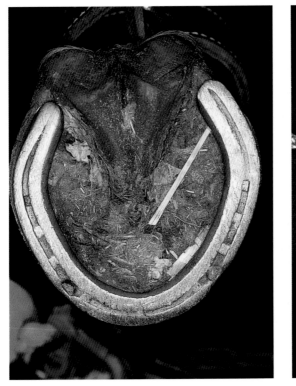

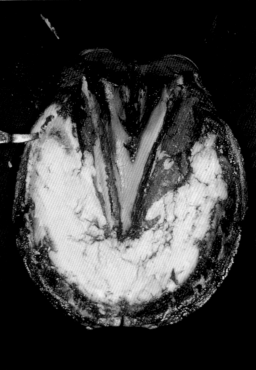

afford it. Insurance is well worth having to cover this eventuality. It is better to know that your horse can have the veterinary care he *needs* rather than only what you can *afford*.

It is essential to have third party insurance cover if you own or ride a horse. Please ensure that you are fully covered as personal injury claims can amount to enormous sums of money.

Left: This shoe has been left on too long, resulting in pressure on the sole at the seat of corn, which will cause lameness

Right: This is a horse with a corn as shown above left, i.e. bruising between the frog and the hoof wall, which has become obvious when the shoe is removed and some of the sole has been pared away

8. HOW TO COPE

It is one thing to read about first aid and another to cope with the situation in reality. Hopefully, by reading this in advance you will be better prepared for most eventualities. No book will be able to prepare you for the harrowing situation of a road accident or something equally ghastly. At the end of the day all you can do is be as calm as you can in the circumstances. Your vet is the best person to advise you, rather than the other onlookers and apparently interested parties, who may interrupt and interfere. To be in control, it helps to know your enemy, i.e. what sort of problem you are dealing with and how serious it may be.

In any emergency, it is essential to prioritise so that first one deals with any life-threatening injury, e.g. by controlling major bleeding. Then sort the non life-threatening but painful conditions, e.g. severe lameness. Then manage the minor injuries and illness, e.g. coughs, cuts and scrapes.

It can be very hard to establish into which category an injured horse should fit. Many horses which are bold and brave when competing can appear to be very distressed and in severe pain with relatively minor injuries. Others, especially some hunters, native ponies and older horses generally, can be very stoical about really major illness. A very careful appraisal is required. If in any doubt, you should always contact your vet.

In human first aid, it is always recommended to consider an ABC, which stands for:

A Airway: i.e. check the patient has a clear airway so that they can breathe.

B Breathing: i.e. check that the patient is actually breathing.
C Circulation: i.e. check that the patient's heart is still beating and that a pulse is present.

This is also worth remembering as a good guideline to use with horses before looking more carefully to try and establish what exactly is wrong.

In an attempt to guide you as to what the problem is, the following lists are included to direct you as to where to look for further information.

What might be wrong if a horse is lying down and cannot stand?

The first thing to check is whether the horse is alive? This may sound patronising but you should think of the ABC above and look:

- to see if the horse is breathing
- if there a pulse or heartbeat
- is there any eye movement? Does the horse blink? If a horse is dead you can touch the eye and there will be no response.

Again, this sort of thing sounds very obvious when written down, yet in the shock of finding your favourite horse flat out it can be harder to remember.

It is rare for a healthy horse to die suddenly with no earlier signs of illness. If this does happen, you should:

- inform your insurers and your vet. The insurance company may require your vet to do a post mortem
- check any other horses kept with the one that has died for signs of ill health
- look for possible causes. The classic cause is electrocution, so make sure all electricity systems in the vicinity are safe.

Once you have established the horse is alive, possible reasons for being unable to stand include:

- azoturia (see page 46)
- the horse being cast (see page 50)
- colic (see page 53)
- collapse (see page 58)
- foaling or problems associated with it (see page 104)
- laminitis (see page 80)
- sudden severe lameness (see page 73)
- shock (see page 92)
- wounds (see page 24).

What could be wrong if a horse is very lame?

You should consider calling your vet immediately if a horse is unable to stand on one leg at all, particularly if he is totally unable to move and appears to be in severe pain. If the lameness is less severe, it is reasonable to rest the horse for a day or so before seeking help from your vet. Your farrier may successfully manage some foot lamenesses.

Look up:

- azoturia (see page 46)
- filled legs (see page 69)
- foreign body in the foot (see page 70)
- laminitis (see page 80)
- sudden severe lamenesses, including fractures, pus in the foot, upward fixation of the patella (see page 73)
- tendon injuries (see page 98).

What could be wrong if your horse is weak, wobbly or reluctant to move?

It can be very alarming if a big horse appears to lose co-ordination and may be about to fall over, or cannot move properly. In most cases it will justify calling your vet right away. Possible causes to look up include:

- azoturia (see page 46)
- colic (see page 53)
- collapse (see page 58)
- haemorrhage e.g. post foaling (see page 117)
- laminitis (see page 80)
- pelvic fractures (see page 116)
- shock (see page 92)
- tetanus (see page 130)
- thumps (see page 100)
- urticaria (see page 87).

What could be wrong if something is draining out of your horse's nose?

This may be either serious or trivial. A major nosebleed must be taken very seriously. However if a horse gets food stuck in its throat (i.e. choke) it can *look* very alarming. Things to look up are:

- breathing problems (see page 48)
- choke (see page 51)
- nosebleeds (epistaxis) (see page 83)
- strangles (see page 94).

How to remove a horse's shoe

This is something which, hopefully, you will never need to do. It is far better to have your farrier do it for you. Ask your farrier if he is available before attempting to do it yourself. However, it is worth watching your farrier carefully and asking him to give you a few lessons just in case you are ever obliged to remove a shoe, for instance, when a shoe has lifted and is pushing on the tender part of the foot. Legally, shoe removal should only be performed by a vet or farrier, unless urgent first aid is required.

If you are going to try and remove a shoe yourself, you do need some strength and expertise. It is also important to have the right equipment and clothing. Leather chaps or a proper farrier's apron are very useful to protect your legs whilst manipulating the horse's foot and pulling off the shoe. You will also need a coarse file, a pair of farrier's pincers (sometimes called pull-offs), a hammer and, ideally, a buffer. In an emergency a pair of DIY pincers would do instead of the proper pull-offs. There are also special first aid purpose-built pieces of kit designed purely to pull off a shoe in an emergency, e.g. the Liveryman Shoemaster®.

To remove a shoe:

1 Lift up the foot and balance it on your thigh, which is a knack in itself. Alternatively, get someone to hold it for you.
2 Rub the wide face of the rasp over the clenches (i.e. nails) several times to rasp them off. If the shoe is still firmly fitted, you may need to use the buffer to lift the nail heads or use a special nail puller.
3 Change position and hold a front foot between your legs or balance a hind limb at a slightly different angle, so that you can start pulling off the shoe. First ease the inside heel of the shoe, followed by the outside. Always pull inwards, towards the frog to avoid breaking the wall of the hoof. This is continued alternately along each branch of the shoe toward the toe until it is loose. Now the shoe can be grasped at the toe and pulled backwards across the foot and off.

4 It may help to pull the raised nails out individually with the pull-offs or pincers. It is possible to have purpose-designed nail pullers to pull each nail head individually away from the shoe.

5 It is of the utmost importance that nails are placed in a bin or special nail box as soon as they are removed, so that the horse does not tread on them.

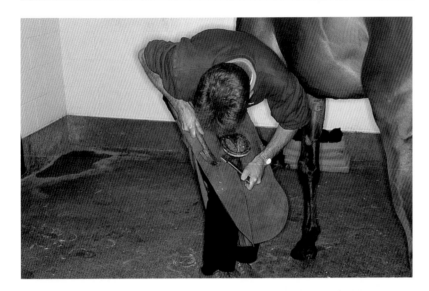

Top: The correct protective clothing is important, so either use a farrier's leather apron as shown, or, better still, ask your farrier or vet to do this for you

Bottom: To lift the clenches from a front foot, the hoof is held between the legs and a farrier's buffer and hammer are used as shown

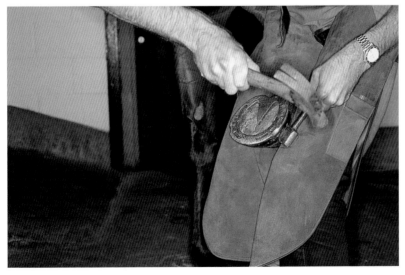

149

Using a pair of
long-handled farrier's
tools (pull-offs) to
remove a shoe after
loosening the nails

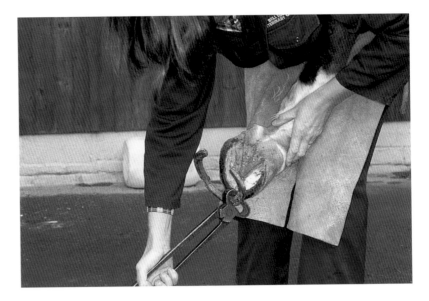

CONCLUSION

Serious disasters are rare. If you are careful and think ahead, you can prevent a lot of problems before they happen. In an emergency it is essential to remain calm. Above all, try to reassure the injured or distressed horse. Unless a general anaesthetic is likely to be required or there is another reason for starving the horse, remember that a filled hay net can work as an effective painkiller. Avoidance of accidents is important. Take sensible safety precautions. This includes ensuring all horses are vaccinated against tetanus. Be prepared to transport the horse to an equine hospital for further investigations and treatment. It is best to consider how you would cope in a crisis before it ever happens, then hopefully it never will. You can then enjoy your horse, safe in the knowledge that you have done everything you can to prepare for and avoid any catastrophe.

USEFUL ADDRESSES AND TELEPHONE NUMBERS

Your own vet:

Your own farrier:

Your own insurance company and details:

Transport if you do not have a box of your own, and to use as a spare if yours is off the road:

The Blue Cross Animal Welfare Charity, Shilton Road, Burford, Oxfordshire OX18 4PF
Tel: 01993 822651
Fax: 01993 823083

British Equine Veterinary Association, 5 Finlay Street, London SW6 6HE
Tel: 020 7610 6080
Fax: 020 7610 6823
E-mail: bevauk@msn.com

The British Horse Society, Welfare Department, British Equestrian Centre, Stoneleigh Park, Kenilworth, Warwickshire CV8 2LR
Tel: 01203 696697

The Home for Rest for Horses, Speen Farm, Lacey Green, Princes Risborough, Bucks HP27 OPP
Tel: 01494 488464
Fax: 01494 488767

The Horserace Betting Levy Board (HRBLB), 52 Grovenor Gardens, London SW1W OAU
Tel: 020 7333 0043

The Humane Slaughter Association, The Old School, Brewhouse Hill, Wheathampstead, Herts AL9 8AN
Tel: 01582 831919
Fax: 01582 831414
E-mail: info@has.org.uk

International League for Protection of Horses, Anne Colvin House, Snetterton, Norwich, Norfolk NR16 2 LR
Tel: 01953 498682
Fax 01953 498373

The Licenced Animal Slaughterers and Salvage Association (LASSA), Unit 4, Chatsworth Technology Park, Dunston Road, Chesterfield, Derbyshire S41 8XA
Tel: 01246 261497

The National Foaling Bank, Meretown Stud, Newport, Shropshire TF10 8BX (membership available)
Tel: 01952 811234
Fax: 01952 811202

The National Rivers Authority, Rivers House, Waterside Drive, Aztec West, Almonsbury, Bristol BS12 4UD
Tel: 01454 624400

Royal College of Veterinary Surgeons, Belgravia House,
62-64 Horseferry Road, London SW1P 2AF
Tel: 020 7222 2001
Fax: 020 7222 2004
E-mail: admin@rcvs.org.uk

The Thoroughbred Breeders Association, Stanstead House,
The Avenue, Newmarket, Suffolk CB8 9AA
Tel: 01638 661321

INDEX

Note: Page numbers in bold refer to figures, those in italics to tables or boxes